# Praise for *A Tired Woman's Guide to Passionate Sex*

"*A Tired Woman's Guide to Passionate Sex* is optimistic about enlivening sex for women who feel that sex is too much work for not enough return! Mintz gives sympathetic advice and easy-to-do tips. I commend the author—and hope women will take advantage of her message. It's never too late to reinvigorate our sexuality."

Pepper Schwartz, PhD
Author of *Prime: Adventures and Advice about Sex, Love, and the Sensual Years*
Past President of the Society for the Scientific Study of Sexuality
President of the Centers for Sexualities at San Francisco State University

"This groundbreaking book is written for all women (and their partners) who have ever been too tired for sex, and who struggle with guilt, shame, resentment, and the loss of sexual desire! Dr. Mintz provides information and guidance in a conversational tone that is honest, humorous, and straightforward. Without a doubt, I will recommend it to my clients, colleagues, friends and relatives!"

Melba Vasquez, PhD, ABPP, Independent Practice, Austin, Texas
Member, American Psychological Association (APA) Board of Directors
Past President, APA Society of Counseling Psychology, APA Society for the
Psychology of Women, and Texas Psychological Association

"*A Tired Woman's Guide to Passionate Sex* should be required reading for all tired women who want to rekindle their sexual desire—and men who want to support them. Basing her work on the best available science, Mintz uses her years of experience as a sex therapist and as a woman to give detailed and wise advice."

Janet Hyde, PhD
Professor of Psychology and Women's Studies, University of Wisconsin
Past President, Society for the Scientific Study of Sexuality
Past President, APA Division for the Psychology of Women
Author of *Understanding Human Sexuality*

"Dr. Mintz takes the woman by the hand and guides her through specific exercises to enhance her sensual and sexual experiences with her partner. A good read for all women who are tired and multitasking."

Beverly Whipple, PhD
Professor Emerita, Rutgers University
Coauthor of *The Science of Orgasm* (2006) and *The Orgasm Answer Guide* (2009)

For more praise, see *www.DrLaurieMintz.com*

# A TIRED WOMAN'S GUIDE TO *passionate* SEX

RECLAIM YOUR *Desire* AND *Reignite* YOUR *Relationship*

LAURIE B. MINTZ, PhD

**ADAMS MEDIA**

NEW YORK  LONDON  TORONTO  SYDNEY  NEW DELHI

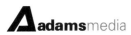

Adams Media
An Imprint of Simon & Schuster, Inc.
100 Technology Center Drive
Stoughton, Massachusetts 02072

For information about special discounts for bulk purchases, please contact Simon & Schuster Special Sales at 1-866-506-1949 or business@simonandschuster.com.

The Simon & Schuster Speakers Bureau can bring authors to your live event. For more information or to book an event contact the Simon & Schuster Speakers Bureau at 1-866-248-3049 or visit our website at www.simonspeakers.com.

ISBN 978-1-60550-107-9
ISBN 978-1-4405-0436-5 (ebook)

Printed in the United States of America.

2 2023

Library of Congress Cataloging-in-Publication Data has been applied for.

# Contents

This book is dedicated to my clients. Thank you for sharing your experiences, thoughts, and feelings with me. Thank you for the honor of being part of your growth and healing.

# Acknowledgments

Although I sat at my computer alone, this book was not a solo-act. This book would not have been possible without the support, advice, and assistance of many people. Writing about sex is easy compared to adequately expressing my gratitude to the people who helped make this book possible.

The people who deserve the utmost gratitude are the ones that need to remain nameless: the women who allowed me to use their stories in this book. Thank you for allowing me to use the intimate details of your lives to help change the lives of others.

Special thanks go to Ali Balzer, my research assistant. Your incredible attention to detail assured the accuracy of every study and statistic cited. In addition, our time working together was a pleasure!

Thanks go to my agent, Jack Scovil. You made the publication of this book possible through your enthusiasm and perseverance. Similar gratitude goes to my editors at Adams Media, Paula Munier and Wendy Simard. Your enthusiasm for the topic and your keen vision both made this book possible and improved its appeal and quality.

This book began many years before I had an agent or an editor. Almost ten years ago, Mary Kay Blakely agreed to help me learn how to adapt my academic writing to the popular press and in the process edited a personal essay about my experience with low sex drive. This essay became the foundation for this book. Mary Kay also gave graciously of her time to help me make a videotape when Adams Media was considering signing me on as an author. Thank you, Mary Kay, for helping me at these two critical junctures of when I wanted to learn to write differently and when I wanted to publish this book.

Two other author-friends deserve much gratitude. Thanks go to Mike Stadler for teaching me about what goes into a book proposal and supporting my initial efforts at writing one. Everlasting appreciation goes to Steve Weinberg, who provided tangible and emotional support every step of the way. Steve, you showed me the kindness of a stranger by taking me under your wing in my book writing endeavor and became a cherished friend in the process.

I am lucky to have friends who not only enrich my life by their presence in it, but who supported me in writing this book. To Karen Rivo, thank you for the conversation that convinced me that I had something book-worthy to say. To Eve Adams and Susan Kashubeck-West, thanks for the conversations about sex that added laughter to my life and enhanced my enthusiasm to write this book. To Cathryn Pridal, thanks for all the times you told me I could do this, even when I didn't believe it myself. Thanks also for the many hours you spent talking and reading, in order to allow me to benefit from your deep bank of scientific and clinical knowledge on the topic of sex therapy. To my peer supervision group and dear friends, Shelly Ossana and Debbie Wright, thanks for your patience when I needed to take a several month furlough from our group, your clinical advice, and your help with the final parts of this book. Several treasured friends were willing to read either chapters or the entire draft of this book and give honest feedback; my gratitude goes to Luanne Andes, Judith Goodman, and Anne Jacobson. Thanks also go to Jessica Middleton and Holly Smith-Berry, once strangers and now women I look forward to continued connection with, for reading this book in its entirety and giving me enormously helpful feedback.

Two very special people also read every word I wrote (sometimes in multiple drafts) as I was writing and gave extraordinarily helpful feedback along the way. To my sister and best-friend-for-life Sari Mintz, thank you for making time in your very busy schedule to read my drafts. Thanks also for all the intimate talks, throughout our lives, about sex and everything else. My mother, Renee Mintz, has been both my most enthusiastic cheerleader and my most honest critic, making me a better person and this book a finer product. It is an understatement to say this book wouldn't have happened without you. Thank you for the vast time you spent and your wholehearted investment in editing drafts. It was obvious that you cared about this book as much as I did! Even more fundamental, I thank you for raising me to believe that I could have a career and a family. Thank you for raising me to believe I could achieve my dreams. Thank you for raising me to believe that sex is something I should enjoy fully and be comfortable talking about. This book represents the intersection of all of these teachings. And, Dad, I smilingly say that except for the latter of these three messages, all this gratitude goes to you too. Talking with you more deeply and more honestly about sex and life in general has been a highlight of these last few years.

To my wonderful daughters, Jennifer and Allison, thank you for putting aside whatever concerns you might have had, and saying you were okay with me writing a book about sex. By doing so, you helped me to pursue my dreams, something I most fervently hope that both of you do in your lives. Thank you for putting up with me sitting for unending hours with my laptop at the kitchen table, trying to strike a balance between being there with you and writing this book—sometimes not too successfully and not too graciously I am sure! Most of all, thanks for always being the joys of my life who I love beyond words.

And, to the love of my life and soul-mate, Glenn Good, thank you for both supporting my dreams and being a grounding force in my life. If you could teach the husbands of all the tired women in the world how to effectively and openly talk with their wives, as well as how to spend time with them, encourage their self-care, touch them, and have trysts with them, this book would be unnecessary. Thank you for living the advice of this book with me. Thank you for helping this tired woman to enjoy both true love and passionate sex.

# Introduction from a Formerly
# Too-Tired Woman and Therapist

You are not alone. At least 33 percent of women say they have lost interest in sex.

The story of my own vanished (and now thankfully regained) sex drive began with motherhood. Both my professional ambition and my sex drive exited with my placenta. Regaining work motivation was a slow yet steady climb up a well-paved mountain. Recapturing my interest in sex has been like a drive down a rocky road, sometimes with no map in hand and other times, with contradictory ones.

After the birth of my first daughter, sex was undeniably less interesting than sleeping or holding her. Still, my second pregnancy is evidence that my husband and I did have intercourse occasionally. For months after my second daughter was born, I felt desperately tired. Between nursing a baby and tending a toddler through nightly asthma attacks, I entered each morning like a red-eye passenger to an undesirable location. When I went back to work, things got worse. My body exhausted and mind preoccupied with guilt, the only time I thought about sex was when I realized I "should do it soon" so my husband wouldn't become too dissatisfied.

He was patient and understanding. As a psychologist, he knows that most new mothers are as motivated toward sex as seven-year-olds are to broccoli. He took solace in jokes by other new fathers about the shortage of passion in their marriages. Still, he said, "I will start to worry if it goes on like this for too long." It did.

One day my husband left a newspaper article on my desk, the first he'd clipped in our twelve years together. The article described how a diminished sex drive in women is often due to low testosterone. A few pills or some cream and WHAM: back comes the lust! Glenn leaving me this article gave me a combination of shame and hope. It was as if a trusted friend had said, "I can really tell that you've gained weight—especially in your butt. But, don't worry! I just heard of a great new diet."

I went to see my doctor. Refusing my request for instant sex drive cream, she told me that my missing passion was a classic symptom of thyroid deficiency. Although recently diagnosed, I had been ill for years. A well-trained psychologist, I attributed depression, anxiety, and exhaustion to my psyche; that the problem was medical didn't occur to me until things were totally out of control. My trusted healer told me, "As soon as your thyroid levels stabilize and your body recovers from the war it fought, you will be as good as new." (I secretly hoped she meant, "You'll feel horny again.")

Potential cure in hand, I began confessing my vanished desire to my closest confidants. "So, what's my problem then?" Eileen, a thirty-five-year-old accountant and the mother of two children, wondered aloud as she confessed that her sex drive was nonexistent. Eileen told me that she tried to have sex once a week or so and that she even enjoyed it once underway. Explaining further,

Eileen lamented, "It's just that I don't have any innate interest anymore. All the hours I have in bed, I absolutely need for sleeping." Andrea, a thirty-six-year-old executive secretary and also the mother of two young children, expressed similar sentiments, telling me that her husband's sexual desire felt like her office phone ringing at the close of the workday. "Sometimes I walk out the door without answering it and sometimes I begrudgingly answer it—fighting resentment and trying to be pleasant—while longing to go home." Sandra, a forty-year-old nurse and mother of young children, rushed to her doctor to confirm that her own thyroid disorder was the culprit for her missing desire. "Decreased sexual energy is not related to currently treated thyroid disorders," Sandra's doctor explained. This physician blamed Sandra's lack of sexual energy on being the mother of a small child—an affliction only many years could cure. Also a mother of small beings, the doctor implored Sandra to "Let me know if you find any solutions!"

> *It's just that I don't have any innate interest anymore. All the hours I have in bed, I absolutely need for sleeping.*
> —Eileen, 35

## A Possible Solution

Fortunately, my doctor had offered a potential solution: Scheduled Sex. As busy and tired and physically rundown as I was, she said I shouldn't wait to be interested in sex. Instead, I should make it a priority and schedule it. "Decide your ideal frequency with Glenn and then schedule times you can have sex each week. Make it part of your weekly schedule."

I discussed the idea with confidants. My friend, Elyse, a therapist specializing in couple counseling, agreed with my doctor. Sandra was also sure the idea of scheduled sex "made total sense." She recited her daily and weekly schedule to me, trying to find times that would work. She discussed our conversation with her husband. Buying into the myth of unplanned passion, he found the idea horribly unromantic. Two weeks later he conceded that sex on a schedule was better than no sex at all.

Glenn didn't take two weeks to decide this. As soon as I discussed the idea of planned sex with him, he was ready to implement a schedule. Since I like sex in the morning and since Glenn feels the opposite, we agreed on one morning and one evening each week.

It worked! Scheduled sex immediately relieved tensions. I didn't need to worry every night as we crawled into bed that Glenn would want sex and I would feel too tired. On our non-sex nights, I could crawl into bed guilt free and get the sleep I needed. On Wednesdays, I stored up my energy and ended up eagerly awaiting sex. And, bluntly, the scheduled sex we had was great sex. Importantly, this regular, good sex resulted in deeper trust and more relaxed and spontaneous laughter. I felt better about myself and my marriage.

At this point, you may be thinking, "So, if it is as easy as planning sex, why the whole book? Why not just tell me to schedule sex and be done with it?" It is because it isn't that easy—not for me, not for my therapy clients, and likely not for you. While scheduling sex was the first step to getting my and Glenn's sex life back on track, it didn't solve the problem of my lost libido. I had sex twice a week and enjoyed it, even having orgasms, but I still never felt spontaneously horny. Years went by and my energizing tingle was gone.

## A Real Solution

Because I wanted to have more than good sex—I wanted to feel horny again—my search for resolution continued. My search was that of a woman seeking relief. I read self-help books and continued my discussions with confidants. I read professional works and consulted with colleagues who specialize in the treatment of sexual problems. I tried ideas promoted by experts and some worked and some didn't. Some recommended strategies that worked were erotic books and increasing the affectionate touching between me and my husband. Still, the strategies I found in both the self-help and professional books were not enough to fully and consistently recover my desire.

Eventually, I realized that this was because none of these strategies focused on the root of the problem. Specifically, none focused on what the majority of women report as the reason for their diminished desire; none focused on exhaustion and stress or on the toll these take on women and their marriages. So, I began "treating" myself with a combination of the best sex therapy strategies AND the most psychologically sound stress reduction strategies. Because of my training as a psychologist, I was also able to effectively communicate my stress-related and sexual needs to my husband. The end result was that I recovered my drive. Importantly, I have been able to continually rely on and come back to these strategies to keep my drive alive, through the inevitable ups and downs of life and of marriage.

As I recovered my sex drive, I passed my combination of strategies to friends who were struggling to recover theirs. Since my method worked, these friends passed my techniques to other women. Word slowly spread, and soon I started receiving professional referrals of women and couples struggling with sexual problems. Now, like many psychologists, I help clients deal with a problem that I overcame myself. I help tired women recover their passion. Now my goal is to help you.

At the start of this chapter, I told you that my road to recovered passion was rocky and unpaved. My purpose is to pave the road for you and make it an easy walk. Let's get started.

*Chapter 1*

# Your Path to Passion

Did you used to have a healthy sex drive but now wonder, "Where did it go and how can I get it back?" If you are among the astonishingly large group of women whose chief complaint is that chronic fatigue and stress from balancing multiple demands has led to a disinterest in sex, this book is designed to help you. The goal of this book is to get you feeling sexual again!

There are nine chapters in this book, including this one. In Chapter 2, I share statistics on the high frequency of decreased sexual desire in women. I explain the multiple possible causes for diminished desire, highlighting the most frequent cause—stress and exhaustion. In order to make sure that this is the reason for your diminished desire, I provide examples of real life women and ask you questions. While I assume you picked up this book because the title resonated with you, I want to make sure that the primary reason for your loss of desire is indeed fatigue and if not, to steer you in the right direction. Then, in Chapter 3 you will learn about the physical, psychological, and relationship benefits of having a good sex life. Starting with Chapter 4, we will get into the "meaty" chapters—the ones that include strategies to help you recover your sex drive.

# Five T's and a Bit of Spice

Chapters 4 through 9 provide what I have found to be an effective and comprehensive six-pronged program for tired women to regain passion. This program combines sex-therapy, marriage enhancement, stress-management, communication skills, and self-care. While admittedly a bit gimmicky, I affectionately call my approach *"Five T's and a Bit of Spice"* and also speak of the *"Five T's for Tired Women."* The *Five T's* are: *Thoughts, Talk, Time, Touch,* and *Trysts.* Akin to a food plan, the *Five T's* are the main course that fulfills your hunger—or in this case, gets you hungering again. The spices are what you add in, according to your taste, to liven up your sex life even further.

The first *T, Thoughts,* is to get you thinking about sex, in positive terms. This step is for you to put positive sexual thoughts on the front-burner of your busy brain, as well as to help you turn off this busy brain during sexual encounters. The second *T, Talk,* is to learn to communicate effectively, both in general and about sex specifically. In my therapy practice, I consistently find that teaching clients a few uncomplicated but elegant communication strategies changes their lives for the better. Thus, the *Talk* step is focused on providing you with these basic strategies. This step is foundational, and you will use the skills that you learn here during the subsequent steps.

The next two *T's* are *Time* and *Touch.* During the *Time* step, you will evaluate what is important to you and will commit to spending more time on these activities, while spending less time on draining, obligatory activities. During the *Time* step, you will be instructed to spend nonsexual affectionate time with your spouse, as well as time organizing the tasks of life together. During the fourth T step, *Touch*, you will learn some straightforward but amazingly effective touching techniques to ignite passion.

Before moving on to the final and most sexually erotic T step of all, *Trysts*, you will have the chance to add some spice to your sex life. Chapter 8 explains how adding something new to your sexual routine can enhance your motivation to have sex. This chapter provides a collection of novel ideas to enliven your sex life and also includes detailed descriptions of what real women who are tired do in the bedroom. I hope this will help you feel more comfortable with sex in all its varieties. Of course, not all of the ideas in these pages will appeal to you and I urge you to listen to your own inner compass about what you like sexually and what you don't.

After working through the first four T's and exploring a few zesty ideas, you will be ready for the final T. My doctor's initial idea of scheduled sex dates has morphed into the most sexually erotic T of all: *Trysts*. You will read about a variety of trysts, ranging from going on a weekend getaway to surprising your partner with hot sex that you have prepared for all day but for which he is caught deliciously off-guard. *Trysts* are a surprisingly little known but extremely effective technique for tired women to rekindle desire. *Trysts* work best when the skills of thinking, talking, taking time, and touching are already in place, and when you have some exciting new ideas that you are interested in trying out. I am hopeful that you will benefit from having *Trysts* be the pinnacle step in your path to passion.

## Walk the Path Together

*The Five T's and a Bit of Spice* method is for women in relation-ships. This is because low sexual desire is something that gener-ally occurs within the context of a long-term relationship. Also, because the vast majority of low-desire women are married, I use the word "husband." For example, I might say, "Talk with your husband about…" or "Do this exercise with your husband." Cer-tainly, there are many women who are not married but who are in long-term relationships that have this same problem; if you are one of these women, I hope you will look past my use of the term husband and fill in the word or name that fits for you.

As you read this book, you might notice that I left culture, race, and religion out, even though many of the real-life exam-ples are from women-of-color and from women from a variety of religious groups. The intersection of race, culture, religion, and sexuality deserves more attention, as do issues of sexuality for women with disabilities. Nevertheless, this book is geared to address as wide an audience as possible: heterosexual coupled women who, regardless of their race, culture, economic status, religion or age, currently feel too tired for sex and who want to find passion once again.

## Getting as Much Passion as Possible from the Plan

There are a few general explanations and instructions that will help you get as much out of this book as possible. Following these instructions is going to increase your chances of feeling horny once again.

## Read It All and in Order

You may be tempted to skip over the initial chapters and go directly to the technique chapters. You might think, "I know my problem is exhaustion so I won't read Chapter 2" or "I already know sex is good for me, so I will skip Chapter 3." Please don't skip the opening chapters. They lay the groundwork to make sure that you will benefit as much as you can from this book.

Along with reading these opening chapters, please read each of the technique chapters in order. If you do this, you will progress from thinking to talking to taking time to touching, and finally—to having erotically electrifying trysts that include some pleasurable new activities.

## Focus on More Than Your Genitals

It is important for you to realize that not all of the techniques you will read about and try will be sexual. In fact, some are not sexual at all. You will especially find much nonsexual material in the *Talk* and *Time* steps. To illustrate, you will be encouraged to talk with your husband about your general needs. Learning to ask for your needs to be met about nonsexual matters will help you recover your sex drive in two ways. First, your needs will be better met so you won't be as depleted, giving you more energy for sex. Second, learning to ask for your needs to be met in nonsexual arenas will help you learn to ask for them to be met sexually. Likewise, in the *Time* step you will be encouraged to spend nonsexual, connected time with your spouse and will be asked to start spending time exercising. Although neither activity is sexual, both are widely known among psychologists as activities that enhance women's sex drive. Women who have lost their sex drive due to stress and exhaustion are particularly in need of strategies that address these root causes.

If you are too tired to have sex, you will need to address both your exhaustion and your sex drive. Your sex drive is part of your life, and not just something that occurs in your clitoris and vagina. This book does not take a genital approach to sex. It takes a whole-person approach, of which your genitals are just one part.

## Sex Is More than Intercourse

Just as sex involves more than just your genitals, your genitals need a lot more than just intercourse. While in popular language the word *sex* has become synonymous with intercourse, sex is much more than penetration. For most women, penetration is not a sexual act that consistently results in orgasm. So, in this book, *sex* is meant in a broader way than intercourse. When referring to intercourse, this word will be used specifically. An important exception is when real women are quoted. In this case, the women's words have not been altered, even if they use the word *sex* to refer to intercourse. Another exception is in Chapter 3, which discusses research on the physical health benefits of sex; most researchers who report these benefits use the word *sex*, even when one might guess that they mean a specific sexual activity such as intercourse. So, when describing these studies, the word *sex* is used except in those rare cases where researchers actually mention a specific sexual act such as intercourse. It is striking that even scientists fall prey to the notion that sex is synonymous with intercourse. As you read this book, remember that sex involves so much more than this one specific sexual act.

## Do Your Homework and Don't Hurry

Throughout this book, you will be given exercises to undertake. Reading this book and expecting it to make a difference without doing the exercises is akin to assuming you will lose weight by paying money to join Weight Watchers, but not following the diet. There is no quick fix for diminished desire. You lost your desire over a period of time, and it will take time to regain it.

You are more likely to regain and hold onto your desire if you absorb this book slowly. Much of the information is best digested in chunks. This is why I often give exercises and then ask you to put the book down and try that exercise for a week. This also mimics the homework given in therapy.

You are rushed and stressed in the rest of your life, and this book is not going to work if you approach it as one more thing to do quickly. As you will learn in Chapter 4, to enjoy sex you need to slow down and revel in the physical sensations. Likewise, to benefit most from this book, you need to unhurriedly take in the information and try the strategies. If you rush through this book by skipping exercises or doing the exercise in less time than suggested, you simply won't get as much benefit as you could.

## Don't Become Disheartened

Some of you will resonate more with one portion of the program than others. For example, the sexual fantasies encouraged in the *Thoughts* step might get Amy's juices flowing again, but do nothing for Sally. Perhaps one of the ideas presented in the *Touch* step will begin to revive Sally's desire; perhaps Sally will feel a much-awaited throb of desire when her husband covertly rubs her inner thigh under the table the way he used to do. Try each of the steps but do not become disheartened if each and every step does not result in immediate effects. Keep on reading and keep on trying, and also remember that these strategies are tools for life that you can continue to come back to in order to keep your sex drive alive.

It is my sincere hope that each and every one of you will finish reading the book with your sex drive back, but I know this isn't realistic. As a psychologist with more than twenty years experience doing therapy, I know that problems are often more complex and multilayered than they initially seem. So, I must say at the outset that a few of you will complete the book without fully recovering your drive. A few of you may be starting this book thinking that your problem is being too tired for sex, and may find out that you have other issues contributing to your low desire. If this is the case, I will point you in other directions for seeking help. Appendix A explains how to find a good therapist and Appendix B recommends self-help books on a variety of topics. Even if you end up discovering that you need additional help for problems not addressed by this book, I am certain that what you learn here will give you the leg-up in dealing with these other issues.

## The Women You Will Meet

I use genuine examples from both friends and clients throughout this book. These people gave me their permission to use their stories—with the promise I would protect their identities. Thus, the names used are never real ones. At times, I change details to further conceal my sources. None of the examples are changed to the point of inaccuracy. My goal was to keep their identities anonymous while maintaining the integrity of each point or situation. My profound thanks go to the people who allowed me to depict the private details of their lives so that I could assist you.

# We're Working Together!

I have written this book as if I were talking with you in my private therapy office. As you read this book, I want you to feel as if you are having a personal and useful talk with someone that you trust. In keeping with this conversational tone, when I tell you about research studies and expert opinions, I say "A study found" rather than saying "In 2008, researchers Smith and Jones found." If you are interested in locating or checking the studies or sources cited, a complete listing by chapter is available on my website (*www.DrLaurieMintz.com*). Along these same lines, I won't use jargon in talking to you through the pages of this book. I will converse with you openly and honestly, in straightforward terms.

I will give you information and advice. I will ask questions to help you pinpoint the issues you are struggling with. I tell my therapy clients that we will work as a team, with my job being to provide information and expertise and their role being to provide the effort needed to think and act differently. The same applies here; together, we will work to help you recover your desire.

*Chapter 2*

# What Zapped My Zeal?

Let's make sure that the reason you have lost your desire is the one that this book addresses: stress and exhaustion from balancing multiple demands. Perhaps you are thinking that you already know this is your problem or else you wouldn't have bought this book. Sometimes, though, people seek help for one problem only to discover that the problem they are seeking relief for is actually a symptom of a different problem. Let's make sure that this isn't the case for you. It probably isn't, but it's best to be sure.

## Understanding Diminished Desire

To understand diminished desire, both the words "desire" and "diminished" have to be defined. To desire sex is to yearn for sexual activity and stimulation. In everyday language, it is to feel horny. Sometimes people say "I'm in the mood" to signify they are desirous of sex. The word "diminished" is important, because it signifies that you don't have something at the same level that you once did.

Diminished desire means you used to have a yearning for sex and now you rarely or never do. Many women describe their loss of sex drive as a lost part of themselves. They lack something they once had, which is what makes diminished desire different from a steady state of never craving or liking sex in the first place. Women who never liked sex can derive some benefit from this book, but it isn't really intended for them. It is for those of you who used to yearn for and seek out sexual pleasure and now don't.

### What Women Say

When describing their diminished desire, some of the things women have told me are:

- *I've gone from a woman of passion to a woman of obligation.*
- *I'm never in the mood anymore.*
- *It's good once it gets going, but I don't have any innate interest anymore.*
- *I don't care if I ever have sex again, but the problem is that my husband still does.*
- *I never think about sex anymore and I used to think about it a lot.*
- *I rarely feel horny, but I make myself have sex with Jim. I feel better after.*

What these women are saying is that their physical sensations of sexual longing are gone altogether or perhaps only rarely and briefly felt.

### A Fleeting Feeling

Jean, a forty-nine-year-old woman with one high school son and a ten-year-old daughter with special needs says "Sometimes I feel horny. But, it's rare and at random moments. And, it's never because I am getting into bed at night." Deborah, a similarly aged woman, describes her desire as a "fleeting whim . . . a dream that vaporizes when you wake up in the morning but try to recall." Deborah says that she "might even have a sensation in my south central region but it is like a twenty-second sound bite. It never lasts long enough to change from whim to intent." Part of this, Deborah says, is because it "takes too much work to get from point A to point B."

This sentiment was echoed by Rebecca, a woman who occasionally wants to act on her fleeting sensations of desire. Her problem however is that "I'm so tired that sometimes it is just easier to take care of it myself." When Rebecca does occasionally feel horny, she doesn't have the kind of energy that she needs for a sexual encounter with her husband, so she masturbates. "I can get there in two minutes" she says. And, besides, there is "no fuss, no foreplay, and it's always good." Still, Rebecca knows that ceasing sexual relationships with her husband is a slippery slope that will harm her marriage.

### No Feeling at All

While Rebecca and Deborah both have occasional, momentary feelings of desire, many women for whom this book is intended simply never experience the pleasant and motivating throbbing, wet ache of desire. They remember feeling this way, and they miss feeling this way, but it is gone. "My libido isn't low—it's nonexistent" says Cynthia, a forty-eight-year old business woman and mother of two. "Sometimes I can't even remember what it used to feel like. It's like that part of me is totally dead" laments Cynthia. Diminished desire is an endless state of not being in the mood.

*My libido isn't low—it's nonexistent.*
—Cynthia, 48

### Sex for Obligation

Because women who are suffering from diminished desire either rarely or never long for sex, they generally don't initiate sex to gratify their own longings. Instead, it is initiated by their husbands and reluctantly agreed upon by them out of a sense of duty or obligation—although it may be quite good once it gets going.

### It's Upsetting

Two studies found that some women who lose their sex drive say they aren't bothered by this. A sexual problem is only a problem if is concerning. My assumption is that you are reading this book because you are troubled by your diminished sexual desire. You aren't satisfied just having sex, even good sex, out of obligation. You used to yearn for and seek out sexual pleasure, and now you don't. This is upsetting to you, your husband, or both of you. You want to feel the way you used to.

# You Are Not Alone:
# The Epidemic of Lost Desire

One hopefully comforting thing to know is that you are not alone. Some surveys report that as many as 52 percent of women say their sex drive isn't what it used to be. Others put the percentages between 20 and 47 percent. The most comprehensive survey conducted to date included a representative sample of the U.S. population between the ages of eighteen and fifty-nine. This study found that 33 percent of women were suffering from a loss of sexual desire. Another well-done study found that one-third of partnered women in the fifty- to seventy-year-old age group had little or no sex drive. That means that one of every three women you know no longer feels as interested in sex as she used to feel!

No wonder that concern about diminished desire is the #1 problem brought to sex therapists. Women also talk to their physicians about their lost desire. My own primary care doctor told me that at least three times each day, one of her patients broaches this topic. My gynecologist tells me that he has a conversation about low or no sex drive about ten times a day! Diminished desire may be epidemic among women.

# No Magic Pill for Diminished Desire

While a multitude of women struggle with a lack of sex drive, there is no magic pill that women can take. While Viagra addressed the most common sexual issue men face, erectile dysfunction, researchers continue to search for a pill to fix women's most common sexual issue, diminished desire. For premenopausal women, some claim success with the antidepressant bupropion hydrochloride

(Wellbutrin). Still, most of the search for a chemical solution focuses on hormones.

## Looking to Hormones

The search for a chemical solution is based on the role of hormones in sexual desire. Hormones are usually classified as male and female, depending on which sex has a higher level of it in their bodies. But, both sexes produce both types. One female hormone, estrogen, helps us maintain vaginal lubrication and elasticity, and also has mood-elevating properties. Its role in sexual desire beyond these effects is unclear. What *is* certain is that the male sex hormones, particularly testosterone, have an effect on our (as well as men's) sexual desire.

## No Risk-Free Hormone Treatment

Livial is a drug that combines testosterone, estrogen, and progesterone (another female hormone). Some studies show it is effective at increasing libido in women. However, at least one study showed that it increased the risk of strokes among women. Livial is only sold in Europe and the United Kingdom; it isn't currently approved by the Food and Drug Administration (FDA).

At the time this book is being written, testosterone gels and patches are also not approved by the FDA for use in women. But, clinical testing is underway, and some findings indicate that a small dose of testosterone applied daily to the upper arm as a gel or patch increases desire among women. Eventual FDA approval seems likely. Before this approval occurs, doctors can legally prescribe testosterone gels and patches "off-label." Off-label prescribing is when a medicine approved to treat one disorder (in this case, men's low testosterone-related problems) is given to treat another for which it hasn't been approved (in this case, women's low sexual desire). Along with testosterone gels and patches, another hormone-based medicine prescribed off-label for low sexual desire is *Estratest*, a combined estrogen-testosterone pill approved for menopausal symptoms such as hot flashes.

While some physicians applaud these testosterone-based pills, gels, and patches as an important breakthrough to help women regain sexual desire, others warn of side effects. Reported side effects include hair growth, acne, and liver damage. Research has shown that testosterone patches might increase the risk of breast cancer when used for just a year.

DHEA is another male hormone. It is available as an over-the-counter supplement. At least one small study supports it positive effect on women's libido. Still, because it generally converts to testosterone in our livers when taken orally, doctors warn it likely has some of the same problems as testosterone. Some point out that it is even less well-studied than prescribed testosterone.

## Another Under-Studied Antidote

Another over-the-counter pill that women sometimes take to increase sexual desire is Argin Max. This nutritional supplement has at least two studies supporting its positive effect on sexual desire. Still, physicians suggest caution when taking this and other over-the-counter supplements because side effects aren't well-studied. Doctors also worry that some women take these supplements before checking into possible interactions with medicines currently being taken.

Clearly, no one has found a pill, gel, or patch that increases women's libido without causing other problems. In addition, some say that even the act of searching for a medical solution to women's low sexual desire is a problem.

## A Misplaced Focus

Some experts express worry that searching for a magic pill will turn women's sexual desire into a medical problem. They are concerned that this will take the focus away from the most common culprits of diminished desire in women, including lack of information on how our own bodies work, body image issues, relationship issues, and a stressful lifestyle, to name just a few. As you know, this latter cause—sheer exhaustion and stress—is the focus of this book.

## Try a Cup of Warm Milk First

Since addressing your stress and exhaustion isn't going to have any dangerous medical side effects, a prudent approach is to engage in the psychological treatment that this book offers before turning to hormone supplements to address your problem of low desire. If you finish this book and still have no sex drive, then you might want to consider a chemical solution. If you do, approach this as a well-informed consumer and advocate for your health. Be aware of the possible side effects and health risks of these treatments. The Appendix B: Additional Resources section points you in directions for more information.

Further reading is likely to make you more keenly aware of the widely mixed opinions surrounding hormone therapy for diminished desire. As aptly stated in a 2004 *New York Times* article by Dr. Susan Love, "If you're confused—it means you've been listening." Dr. Love goes on to say, "With testosterone patches for women with low libido on the horizon, we should be asking how much we really know about their long-term safety. . . . We need to realize that we are making decisions on the use of hormones based on inadequate information."

You don't have to take that risk with this book. The treatment offered in this book is based on time-tested psychological principles. There are certainly no known negative medical side effects associated with good communication or spending time with your spouse! Trying this book before taking hormones is akin to taking a hot bath and drinking a cup of warm milk for insomnia before turning to sleeping pills. Before addressing what may be a lifestyle issue with a pill, let's address the lifestyle issue itself: being too tired for sex.

## Too Tired for Sex

Being too tired is the #1 reason that women blame for their loss of desire. A great number of women say that their primary issue is being too depleted to have interest in sex and not some looming issue such as hating one's husband or having been the victim of sexual trauma. While some couples cease having sex due to troubled relationships, women who say that they are too tired for sex are generally happy with their relationships, yet have no sex drive. Still, women who say they are too tired for sex may also have some other issues that cause diminished desire. They may have communication problems with their husbands, or issues with lack of lubrication. But, if asked to say the primary reason for their missing passion, the answer given by countless women is that they are too wiped out to have sex.

Does this description fit you? Do you relate to the notion of not being in the mood and having sex anyway? Is sex sometimes surprisingly satisfying when it gets going? Sometimes, though, is sex less than satisfying because you rush through it so you can get some shuteye? If you answered yes to these questions, you are likely among the vast number of women who are too tired for sex.

### Which Women Are Too Tired for Sex?

Who are all of these women who, like you, feel too tired for sex? Women who feel too tired for sex are generally in their late twenties through early sixties and balancing demands between work, children, and perhaps aging parents. Married women with children who work outside the home seem to be the most likely to report feeling too tired for sex. Still, many women who don't work outside the home also feel too wiped out for sex. These women are depleted and exhausted from caring for their homes and their children, sometimes without their spouse adequately sharing in these responsibilities. Likewise, many women finish raising children and then switch to caring for aging parents or in-laws. Some are sandwiched between both. Women who are too tired for sex come from all walks of life; what they share in common is the feeling that sex takes too much energy—energy that they don't have when they crawl into bed at night exhausted.

## What Is Making You Too Tired for Sex?

What is exhausting you, and all these other women, so much that sex sounds like one more chore to do at the end of a long day?

Caring for others without enough focus on yourself is one reason for feeling too tired for sex. Constant caretaking is a libido zapper. Reveling in sexual sensations and activities requires a complete focus on nothing but oneself, and this means quite a switch if you're used to focusing on others. It is hard to shift from taking care of others to prioritizing your own sexual pleasure. As Ashley, a fifty-year-old woman with three children, summed it up, "The last thing I think of is me. I am so focused elsewhere that for a long time I didn't even notice anything was missing." Women are often so intent on caring for others that they don't have time to care for themselves. Such women are caught in a vicious cycle of too much to do, not enough sleep, and not enough self-focus, leaving them without energy for sex. Women who are depleted and stressed are not going to want to have sex.

> ## *The last thing I think of is me.*
> ### —Ashley, 50

Stress is another driving force behind lost libido. Serious stressors such as the death of a loved one or the loss of a job have been long known to interfere with sexual drive. But, daily stressors destroy libido as well. The experience of vacation sex is illustrative when it comes to the effects of stress on a woman's sex drive. Many women report that while on vacation, without to-do lists and the pressures of daily life, their sex drive returns—only to go into hibernation again when they return home. In fact, it is often such an experience that helps confirm for women that their missing libido is a result of their stressful and busy lifestyle. Have you ever had the experience of regaining your sex drive on vacation only to lose it again when you return home? If so, this is further confirmation that your busy and stressful lifestyle is the reason for your missing passion.

# How Stress Zaps Libido

Just how stress interferes with your sex drive includes both psychological and physiological components. If you are stressed out, you are going to be distracted and thus unable to relax and focus on sex. And, even if you do have sex in this unfocused condition, it is likely to be sex in which your mind is elsewhere. A wandering mind is sure to make sex less than satisfactory. And, having mediocre or bad sex is only going to further decrease your drive. Stress can also contribute to insomnia and there is no doubt that lack of sleep diminishes sex drive.

Another physiological effect of stress is the secretion of cortisol, a fight or flight hormone. As cortisol increases, testosterone, which is responsible for much of our sex drive, decreases.

## Sex Differences: Pig Poop and Dirty Socks

Did you ever wonder why women's sex drives seem to be more affected by stress than men's? The effects of cortisol can help explain this. As you just read, stress results in the release of cortisol, and cortisol decreases testosterone. Men have about ten times more testosterone than women. So, thinking of sex drive as a tank of gas, stress-induced cortisol may take a woman's reserve to empty, yet only decrease a man's tank to half full.

Stated in fancy, technical terms, women experience more "erotic plasticity" than men. Women's sexual moods fluctuate more as a result of external sources than do men's. This is best illustrated by a story my gynecologist tells in response to the ten times a day he hears concern about diminished sex drive from his patients. According to my doctor, a man could be standing knee deep in a pile of pig poop and if an attractive woman walks by, he will think about sex. A woman can be headed to her bedroom ready for a sexual encounter and see a dirty sock on the floor and it's all over!

This is not to say that men don't lose their sex drive due to stress. Research shows that some men report that stress zaps libido. Other men say stress revs up their sex drive. But, for the vast majority of busy, stressed women, sex ends up being perceived as another drain on time and energy. Men, on the other hand, are more likely to complain that their wives are not interested in sex.

## Some Life Stages Feel Sexier Than Others

During some life stages, stress and exhaustion are unavoidable. During such stages, one can expect a decreased libido. Despite popular beliefs, your sexual drive waxes and wanes.

For women who are parenting, sex drive typically follows what researchers call a U-curve. It is high in one's youth and declines during the early parenting years, and then—if the relationship is good—increases again when children get older and particularly when they leave home. Of course, depending on when menopause (average age fifty-two, give or take five years) comes in this life cycle, things may look a bit different. Sex drive generally declines, but also sometimes increases, in menopause. Let's take a look at two life stage issues that can affect sex drive.

### The "Do No Harm" Years of Early Parenting

In a recent survey, 26 percent of new mothers said they were too exhausted for sex. When asked what they would most like to do if it was Saturday night and their baby was asleep, 38 percent said that their first choice would be to sleep. In the words of Jean as she reflected on this stage of her life, "I remember being so totally overwhelmed and exhausted." In addition to sheer exhaustion, hormone changes that occur after giving birth and during breast-feeding can dampen desire; women who are breast-feeding have less vaginal lubrication, and being less wet makes sex less enjoyable. Likewise, changes in body image and the pressures of caring for a new baby contribute to diminishing desire. As stated by Carla, a thirty-three-year-old mother of two children under the age of three, "It's almost as though giving birth just destroyed my sex drive. Greg and I were so passionate when we dated and during marriage before kids. Suddenly it was as though the kids simply replaced our own relationship."

> *It's almost as though giving birth just destroyed my sex drive.*
> —Carla, 33

While this is common, it is a slippery slope. If Carla and Greg let their children replace their own relationship, they may end up with no relationship at all. They may end up like Sally and Anthony, who let their new parenting lack of sex drive spiral out of control; their children are six and eight and they still haven't had sex. Sadly, this is not uncommon; no-sex marriages often begin in the early parenting years.

The early parenting years can be thought of as the "Do No Harm" stage of a relationship. In other words, while it is natural for the focus on both the couple part of the relationship and sex to decrease during these years, enough attention must be paid so that no harm is done to the marital relationship. To do no harm means that you and your partner do enough attending to your relationship that you are still connected to one another. The goal is to make sure you still know and love each other when the breathing room that comes with children growing up occurs, or in the words of Jean you "finally feel like a person again." You must also avoid buying into the myth that children shouldn't change your relationship. Expecting one's marriage and sex life to be the same after-kids as it was before-kids is unrealistic. New parents must strike the balance between knowing that while the focus is on children, their relationship is not going to feel as intimate and primary, and still making sure that it is nurtured.

The techniques in this book will help prevent new parents from losing sight of their sexual relationship. It can aid parents who are experiencing a natural decline in sex drive keep this decrease from turning into a sexless marriage. The techniques can also help those in longer term no-sex marriages. However, lack of sex in a marriage will cause other discord, and depending how deep this knife has already cut, you may end up needing additional help beyond this book. If you find that this is the case when you finish reading, the Appendices will help.

## Menopause and Sex Drive: It Depends

Earlier, I advised that you reject the myth that children shouldn't change your relationship. Another myth that can cause harm is that time and aging shouldn't change our sex lives. Our bodies, and those of our spouses, go through changes as we age. As men age, they typically need more stimulation to get and maintain an erection. As women reach menopause, they often experience vaginal dryness, a topic that will be covered later. While certainly not all perimenopausal and menopausal women experience a decreased libido, many do, and there is some evidence that this is at least partly biochemical. Testosterone, responsible for much of our sex drive, decreases in the forties, the common age of perimenopause. Then, as menopause hits, estrogen also decreases and with it, our natural vaginal wetness. Other symptoms of menopause, such as hot flashes, mood swings, and insomnia, are also libido zappers. Doctors sometimes prescribe estrogen-based hormone therapy to alleviate these symptoms, particularly when they are interfering with a woman's life. Although many women report that such hormone therapy successfully alleviates their menopausal symptoms (and thus perhaps makes them feel more sexual), there is some evidence that orally ingested estrogen can further diminish sexual desire. Also, some large studies have reported side effects, including increased risk for breast cancer, stroke, heart attack, and blood clots.

While hot flashes, mood swings, insomnia, and decreased desire are common complaints among menopausal women, it is important to realize that not all women in this age group experience these symptoms. Some women report that their sex drive increases and sex gets better as they age, perhaps because they better know their own bodies and are less afraid to say what they want and need sexually. Certainly, the very active sex life of many menopausal women tells us that hormones aren't the whole story. The fact that midlife women who have a new sex partner generally report a very high sex drive further demonstrates that other issues besides hormones—such as anger at one's spouse or stress in one's life—also contribute substantially to decreased desire.

# Start Reinventing

Oftentimes, we deny sexually related changes of aging. We understand that we won't see, hear, or remember things as well at sixty as we did at twenty, and consider this "par for the course." However, when it comes to sex, many people expect things to stay the same, despite aging. As aptly stated in an article by Natalie Angier in the *New York Times*, "… many people still yearn to burn more, to feel ready for bedding no matter what the clock says and to desire their partner of 23 years as much as they did when their love was brand new."

Alex, a sixty-three-year-old client, was wondering why his sexual responsiveness wasn't what it used to be. I pointed out that he doesn't wonder why he is bald or his vision isn't what it used to be. Since Alex is an ex-college athlete, I also pointed out that he doesn't expect to compete on the local college swim team at his current age. He laughed and said that he got the point.

The point is that because the newness and intensity of young adult sexuality is so powerful and breathtaking, we pine away for these days. We wonder what is wrong that we don't feel this way anymore, even when we are smart enough to not expect other things to be the same. Mirroring this sentiment, my friend Lydia, a fifty-four-year-old mother of two and teacher at a local middle school, tells me that she "longs for the days when it felt like we invented sex." Kelsey, a forty-seven-year-old client tells me that she wistfully recalls the time in her life when "the very air seemed to have a sexual charge to it." I told Kelsey, and am now telling you, it is rare for women to get back to this state of sexual energy because this life-stage occurred in youth, before being tired out by children, aging parents, bills, medical issues, jobs, household chores, and the like. To set the goal of getting back to a state of constant heightened arousal is likely to result in disappointment. A more reasonable goal is to adjust to your current life stage.

Adjusting doesn't mean accepting one's lack of sex drive and giving up, however. Adjusting means to set reasonable goals and work to accomplish them. A reasonable goal is that you will reinvent your sexuality in a way that fits your current life stage. A realistic goal is that you will again come to desire and enjoy sex in your marriage. A reasonable goal is that the current tension about your lack of sex drive will dissipate. Hopefully, sex will again become an important part of your life. But, before moving on to the treatment program that will help you reach these goals, let's make sure that you aren't overlooking another cause of your diminished desire.

## What Else Within Me Could It Be?

There are many other reasons besides being tired and stressed that cause a loss of sexual desire. More than one woman has told me that she wonders if the reason she has lost her sex drive is that she used up her quota of good sex early in her life! While it is interesting that multiple women have asked this question, it is not a reason for diminished desire. We don't have a lifetime limit on good sex.

There are countless legitimate reasons for diminished desire. To use a metaphor, a woman who has an allergy attack while visiting a relative who has a cat will assume that she is allergic to cats. But, it may be that the allergy isn't really to the cat at all, but to the dust mites that she couldn't see. Or, maybe she is allergic to both cats and dust mites. The same is true of sexual desire. It can be due to exhaustion or to a different reason, or to both exhaustion and this other reason combined. Let's make sure what you are really struggling with is diminished desire from exhaustion and not some other issue for which another source of help would be more useful.

Seeking help elsewhere can mean finding a good physician or psychologist, or it could mean reading a different book. Tips for finding a therapist can be found in Appendix A. Books for other problems, as well as for deeper exploration of some topics in this book, can be found in Appendix B.

## Not Liking Your Body

Being dissatisfied with one's body is a common reason for diminished desire. In a survey of women between thirty-five and fifty-five-years of age, most said that they considered themselves less attractive now than ten years ago. Even worse, almost 21 percent disliked their bodies so much that they could not even name one feature they considered attractive! Perhaps you won't be surprised to learn that women were most dissatisfied with the parts of their bodies that naturally gain weight with age: legs, hips, stomachs, and thighs. Most important, feeling less attractive was highly related to a decreased desire for sex!

This study mirrors my clinical practice. Oftentimes, a woman loses her sexual desire because she is ashamed of her body. But, body shame is not consistently related to weight or body shape. Karen is a divorced thirty-seven-year-old insurance agent and the mother of two young children. Karen's body weight would put her in the obese category. She has a high sex drive. She and her boyfriend meet twice a week for dinner and intensely passionate sex. Bethany, on the other hand, is a normal-weight thirty-two-year-old woman suffering from extreme body hatred. Her comfort with sex fluctuates with her weight; a three-pound weight gain is enough to have her avoid sex. Regardless of actual size, those who feel bad about their bodies are more likely to not want to have sex, or to hide under the covers with the lights off when they do.

Hiding under the covers or avoiding sex isn't necessarily related to your husband's reaction to your body. Candice is a forty-three-year-old stay-at-home mother of two boys. By objective standards, she is slightly overweight. She is deeply ashamed of her body and does everything she can to avoid sex with her husband, Kenneth. Kenneth reports that he loves Candice and is attracted to her. He says that he wants nothing more than to have sex with her. He claims that the only thing getting in the way is her uneasiness with her body. For Candice and Kenneth, then, the only issue is Candice's body shame and not lost attraction in the relationship.

For other couples, lost attraction is the issue; this will be discussed later when describing relational issues that can fuel diminished desire. Lost attraction needs to be dealt with as a couple's issue whereas feeling too fat for sex, despite a husband's reassurances, is an individual woman's issue to deal with. Like women who feel too-tired-for-sex, women who feel-too-fat-for-sex generally report that when they finally get between the sheets, they enjoy sex. What often helps is thinking more positive thoughts and focusing on the pleasure one's body can give rather than what it looks like. Exercise also helps. Both positive thinking and exercise are also prominently featured in this book as ways to help women who are too tired for sex. So, if you have lost your sex drive because you are exhausted and you don't like your body, this book can help. If the only reason your sex drive is in hiding is because of body shame, a book more focused on this issue or therapy will be a more direct route to feeling better.

### Not Feeling Well

Speaking of feeling better—or its reverse, not feeling well—sometimes health issues and medications are the culprit for diminished desire. Feeling unwell physically and feeling sexy don't go together. Jean summed up the issue with a question for which she really didn't expect an answer: "How does one make PMS night sweats sound passionate? Or gas related to lactose intolerance and acid reflux?" Jean was lamenting the fact that there are legitimate health-related reasons for diminished desire.

*How does one make PMS night sweats sound passionate?*

—Jean, 49

Two mental health issues that can zap desire are addictions and depression. Drug and alcohol abuse diminish desire. Depression and some of the medications given to alleviate it diminish libido. Antidepressant medications, particularly serotonin re-uptake inhibitors (SSRIs) such as Prozac and Zoloft, may reduce arousal.

Angela is a woman in her mid-forties who struggles with depression. Without her medication, she has a hard time functioning and spirals down into what she calls "the bad place." So, she takes Prozac to ward off the depression and it works marvelously, but her sex drive is diminished and her ability to orgasm lessened. This is a difficult issue, because these sexual problems are further upsetting to Angela. For now, she has chosen the trade-off of feeling less depressed, although her orgasms "feel like a one on the Richter scale instead of an eight or ten." Because it has fewer sexual side-effects, Angela is contemplating switching to the antidepressant Wellbutrin, but she is understandably hesitant to make this change since her current medicine works well. For now, Angela works to decrease the amount of antidepressant medication she needs by exercising and taking time for herself, things that this book will also put forth as means to increase desire. So, if your diminished desire is due to depression and the antidepressant medications used to treat it, this book won't be the cure-all. But, it will offer strategies that are good for your overall mental well-being and your sexual well-being.

Diminished desire can be an early sign of a potentially serious underlying medical issue. Health issues that can dampen desire include thyroid problems, chronic pain, bladder control problems, arthritis, cancer, diabetes, high blood pressure, neurological diseases, and tumors of the pituitary gland. Cardiovascular disease and hypertension can also decrease libido by reducing blood flow to the entire body, including the genital area. Conditions such as endometriosis and fibroids can also decrease sex drive. Likewise, certain prescription medications affect libido. These include blood pressure medications, tranquilizers, antihistamines, and chemotherapy drugs. Some birth control pills also decrease sex drive, although unfortunately these are also generally the ones with fewer other side effects such as weight gain, headaches, and mood swings.

Given all these potential medical and medication-related reasons for loss of sexual desire, whenever a client comes to me for this concern, I send her to a physician for a complete workup. Every once in a while, a medical issue, such as low thyroid, is discovered. This means that therapy wouldn't have done much good. Perhaps my client would have learned to cope better with her distress, but the underlying medical reason for the distress would still be present.

**CALL YOUR DOCTOR TODAY!**

Please talk to your doctor to see if a health issue or medication is responsible for your lack of sex drive. Many women are uncomfortable bringing up the subject of sexual difficulties with their doctors and according to a survey conducted by the Women's Sexual Health Foundation, more than 90 percent of doctors don't ask. Unfortunately, just because someone has an MD degree doesn't mean they are trained in or comfortable with discussing sexual issues with women. While primary care doctors and gynecologists should ask about sex and intimacy as part of a routine medical visit, if they don't, it is up to you to be your own medical advocate and bring the topic up. Sex is an important part of your physical and emotional well-being and is completely appropriate to discuss with your physician. If your doctor makes you feel like your problem is in your head, you have the right to find a new doctor. Similarly, if your doctor focuses only on your genital symptoms and doesn't ask you questions about your emotional or relational well-being, this is another sign that you need a physician better trained in sexual issues. Your doctor should make sure that your low desire isn't due to a medical issue or medication, such as those mentioned above. Your doctor might also explore your hormone levels; if hormone therapy is recommended, be an informed consumer. Take another look at the earlier section on this topic and see Appendix B for additional readings on the topic. Ask lots of questions, especially about side effects. Feel free to express concerns about such treatments or to discuss waiting to start such treatments until you have finished working on the psychological strategies that this book offers.

I urge you to put the book down right now and go to the phone and schedule a time to see your doctor. You can certainly keep reading this book and doing the exercises while you wait for your appointment.

### Not Sleeping Well

Insomnia, or the inability to fall or stay asleep, is another issue that affects libido. You are not going to feel horny if you are not getting enough sleep. In a recent survey, 58 percent of women said that they were less interested in sex after a poor night's sleep. Consistently not sleeping well can be caused by a multitude of psychological and physiological issues. The difficulty is figuring out what is causing the insomnia and overcoming it.

Stress can cause insomnia. In this case, then, the same thing that causes women too feel too tired for sex causes them to toss and turn all night long. Dianna, a fifty-four-year-old woman with sleep problems, recently realized that "My need for sleep medicine began when sex ended." Dianna is in the process of working through the six steps in this treatment program because she thinks "sex would be a better way to get to sleep again." If, like Dianna, stress is affecting both your sleep and your sex life, this book is for you.

*Sex would be a better way to get to sleep again.*
—Dianna, 54

On the other hand, if there is doubt about what is causing your insomnia, it is best to check it out with a physician. Insomnia can be caused by medications, including those for allergies, high blood pressure, and asthma. Caffeine, alcohol, and nicotine are also associated with sleep disturbances. Certain medical conditions are associated with insomnia such as acid reflux disease, asthma, and heart problems. Many women report insomnia to be a symptom that occurs before or after menopause; sometimes this is due to night sweats and sometimes it is a symptom in and of itself. Also, of course, a partner who snores or sleeps restlessly can contribute to your insomnia. If any of these are issues for you, alleviating them will go far in recovering your sex drive. See a doctor to make sure medications or an illness is not responsible for your insomnia. Cut down on alcohol, caffeine, and nicotine, particularly before bed. If your husband snores or is restless, cajole him to see a physician. A good motivator may be learning that taking care of these issues will improve your sex drive and result in more sex for him!

## Dealing with the Emotional Pain of Infertility

Another issue that can affect sex drive is infertility. Women undergoing fertility treatment often feel their bodies have failed them and intercourse reminds them of this. Intercourse also comes to be thought of as a means to accomplish an elusive but important goal instead of something done for pleasure and connection. These issues can last for years after infertility treatments, even successful ones. If this is the case for you, therapy and support groups can be useful, as can books on dealing with infertility issues. However, the ideas in this book are also likely to help; changing the way you think about sex and spending connected, affectionate time with your spouse can be important steps to recovering your desire for sex.

## Surviving a Sexual Trauma

One reason for a diminished sexual drive that this book won't help with is trauma. Surviving a rape or sexual assault, either in your childhood or adult life, is going to affect many aspects of your life, including your sex life. The best way to heal from such a trauma is to get therapy from an experienced psychologist. Indeed, recovery from trauma is completely possible with good help. If you are the survivor of a sexual trauma, it is likely that your lack of desire stems from this. Please turn ahead to Appendix A and read about locating a good therapist. You will also find some excellent self-help books in Appendix B.

## Having Negative Notions about Sex

Your attitude about sex is critical to your sex drive and enjoyment. Some people don't have a good sex life because they have negative attitudes about sex. Some women have been taught that good girls don't enjoy sex, that sex is dirty, and the like. A therapist I know tells his clients that to enjoy sex they have to first kick out of their bedroom all the rabbis, priests, mothers, fathers, teachers, aunts, uncles, and anyone else who instilled negative attitudes about sex.

Someone who has a positive attitude about sex isn't likely to suddenly acquire a negative one. However, two particular attitudes may fuel diminished desire: attitudes about sex and emotional intimacy, and attitudes about sex and aging.

Amber, a forty-eight-year-old occupational therapist with a seventeen-year-old son says the following about her second husband, who she considers her best friend and soul mate. "My problem is that we are so close, he is like family. I tell him everything and I have bared my soul to him. He is like a brother and it's backfired because you aren't supposed to have sex with your brother." The idea behind Amber's thoughts is that steamy, physical sex with someone we love, respect, and are emotionally intimate with isn't proper, and that sex is a dirty thing best relegated to strangers or people we don't care about. If this, plus exhaustion, describes your thought processes, you can benefit from this book. You will find the *Thoughts* and *Trysts* steps most useful, although it is still recommended that you read the entire book to derive the most benefit.

Attitudes about sex and aging can also be associated with diminished desire. Someone who believes that older people shouldn't enjoy sex or that sex is only for the young is likely to be affected by this attitude when they hit their later years.

In the next chapter we will zero in on your attitudes about sex and try to change them to a more titillating mindset. So, if negative thinking about sex is contributing to your diminished desire, this book can help.

## What about Us Could It Be?

Relationship issues loom large when talking about sexual issues, either because the relationship issues are the root cause of the sexual issue or because the sexual issues have harmed the relationship. While things are not always so clear-cut, it is still useful to think of relationship and sexual issues in this chicken-and-egg manner. If relationship issues are primary, this is what needs to be fixed first, whereas if sexual issues are occurring in the context of a good relationship, the sexual issues need to be the first order of business. This book is aimed at those of you who feel positively about your husband and your marriage, but who are nevertheless uninterested in sex. Still, let's examine relationship issues that can be at the root of sexual problems.

### One or Both of Us Was Unfaithful

Affairs often wreak havoc on marriages. Although some women say that an affair was what helped them rediscover their sex drive, even to the benefit of their marriage, mental health providers wouldn't generally endorse this method of enhancing libido. While perhaps an occasional marriage can escape unscathed by an affair, most are damaged. The damage that is caused by an affair can occur even if the affair remains secret.

Let's take Beth, a thirty-two-year-old woman who had an affair during the third year of her marriage. Beth ended the affair and soon thereafter, lost her sex drive. What happened was that out of guilt and fear of having another affair, Beth shut off all of her sexual feelings. Feelings in general, and specifically sexual feelings, are not something that can be turned selectively off or on. So, when Beth shut off her sexual feelings, she was unable to turn them on again.

The solution is definitely not having another affair to rev up her sex drive, nor is it necessarily telling her husband about the affair since this may cause more damage at this point. What Beth needs to do, perhaps with the aid of a good therapist, is to forgive herself and move forward, allowing sexual feelings to re-enter her life while resolving that she won't have sex outside of her marriage again.

If an affair is at the root of sexual problems, recovery from the affair is the primary issue to be dealt with and not the sexual relationship. For this, a good self-help book is recommended, as is an experienced and skilled couples therapist. If your diminished sex drive is due to an affair you had, one your husband had, or both, skip ahead to Appendices A and B.

## We're Angry and in a Power Struggle

Another common issue that can be at the root of sexual problems is anger and power plays in the marriage. While some individuals report that anger fuels their sex life by increasing emotional intensity and through make-up sex, psychologists agree that this route to passion is not a healthy one. Built up resentments and deep-seated anger are not good for relationships.

Patricia is a thirty-eight-year-old woman who has ceased having sex with her husband. "Why should I give him anything he wants? He is completely unappreciative of all I do and constantly critical of me." Patricia is deeply dissatisfied with her marriage, and using sex as a weapon to get back at her husband for what she perceives as his nastiness. Georgina also punished her husband by withdrawing sexually; she was punishing him for the many long hours he spent at work. Using sex as a weapon is not a healthy choice. Resentments and disagreements are much better off dealt with through direct communication.

*Poor communication is what killed*
*our sexual relationship.*
—Phyllis, 44

### We Don't Know How to Talk about It

Communication problems can themselves be at the root of sexual problems. Phyllis, a forty-four-year-old woman who has not had sex with her husband in over a year, says "There are a lot of reasons, but communication is huge. For me, poor communication is what killed our sexual relationship." According to Brad, a fifty-four-year-old plumber, lack of communication also ruined his marriage. Brad says, "I'm a talker. My first wife wouldn't talk to me about anything, including what she wanted sexually. Men are dumb as doorknobs about how to pleasure a woman. We don't need the same things they do. If she would have told me what she wanted in our marriage and in bed, I would have been happy to do it. But, she wouldn't talk to me and it ruined the marriage." While Brad sees the lack of communication as one-way street (his wife wouldn't talk to him), with most communication problems, both partners contribute.

If exhaustion and stress have zapped your sex drive, and you don't know how to talk with your husband about it, this book is ideal. If you feel deep anger and loathing toward your husband and have little confidence that you could talk this through, this book is not for you. This book will be like putting a band-aid on a cut that needs stitches. It will offer superficial, minimal assistance only. You would be better off getting stitches first, with stitches in this case being marriage counseling. If you fit somewhere between these two scenarios, or are not sure where you fit, give this book a shot. You can always put it down and try couples counseling instead, or in addition to, this book.

## We Don't Feel Attracted Anymore

Another thorny relationship issue that can cause diminished desire is lost attraction. Earlier we talked about women who lose desire because they don't like their own bodies, even when their spouses tell them they are attractive. Lost attraction, on the other hand, is when one spouse finds the other sexually unappealing. Oftentimes, lost attraction is related to a physical change in one spouse, such as weight gain.

Both Judy and Linda are women in their early fifties who report not being attracted to their spouses for the same reason: his bulging belly. Both women love their spouses and have no intention of leaving their marriages; they simply find their husband's physique to be a turn-off. Judy spent several months working up the courage to tell her husband this. When she did, he was responsive. He wanted to be sexually intimate again and said that if his weight was the issue, he would do something about it. He asked for Judy's support and she gave it. They started eating healthily together and taking walks after dinner. Judy took over some of Kevin's early morning child duties so he could go the gym. Kevin lost twenty pounds and Judy's interest returned.

Linda's story isn't so happy. She has repeatedly told her husband, Sal, that until he loses weight, she isn't interested in being sexual with him. Sal agrees that his weight is an issue, but refuses to do anything about it. Sal is choosing food and his sedentary lifestyle over sex and while this is his choice, he can't expect Linda to be happy about it.

If, like Linda, you feel no sexual desire for your spouse due to a physical change in him, then you may have selective rather than generalized diminished desire. A key question to ask is if you feel attraction for other men. If you are sexually drawn to other men, while feeling turned off by your spouse, then you aren't just too tired for sex. You have lost your attraction to your husband. This book isn't going to help. Try individual or couples therapy instead. The same is true if you are the object of your spouse's lost desire due to significant weight gain. As painful as this can be, it is best to deal with it directly. Rather than grumble about how superficial your husband is to care about your appearance, a better approach is to realize that physical attraction is part of sexual desire between couples. A good place to start (and one that will also increase your libido) is with good nutrition and physical exercise.

## We're Bored in Bed

Another issue that can contribute to diminished desire is sexual boredom. Sexually, some people crave dependability, whereas others desire novelty. Laura craves novelty, and Faith gets off just fine with dependability.

For Faith, a fifty-two-year-old bank teller and mother of two, the fact that her husband knows just how to turn her on is more important than doing different things. "We follow the same routine every time. It's like wearing my favorite pair of shoes. I know they will feel great every time. I prefer that to breaking in a new pair, which might give me blisters."

Laura, a similarly aged teacher and mother of eight-year-old twins, feel the opposite. "Part of the reason I don't care if I have sex is because it is so boring. It's the same old thing every time. The rest of my life is so rigidly orchestrated that at least in my sex life, I want novelty and surprises."

Are you bored in bed? Are you downright exhausted most of the time? If you said you are bored but not tired, monotony is likely the issue zapping your sex drive. You may not need this entire book. See Chapter 5 for help talking with your husband about spicing things up, and Chapter 8 for suggestions to do so. If you said you are weary of the same old sexual routine, as well as stressed and exhausted, this book is for you.

## He Isn't Interested

Another issue that sometimes emerges for couples is uneven levels of sexual desire. Some people in this situation advocate that it is the duty of the lower-drive spouse to put out, even when not in the mood. Others proclaim that the lower sex-drive spouse should be in charge of how often sex occurs. More sound expert advice involves communication and compromise. You'll find that here.

This book is geared to those women who have a lower sex drive than their spouses. For some women, lack of sex drive is a result of a husband's lost desire. Hilary, a fifty-six-year-old dance instructor, began to bury her sex drive when her husband lost his. Jim became less interested in sex when he saw her give birth and realized that her vagina had another function. This was a turn-off he has not been able to overcome. Hilary remained interested in sex with Jim, but after years of him not being interested, she turned her feelings off. While raising a young child, this didn't bother her because as she says, "I didn't have much time or energy for sex either, even though if Jim had been interested, I would have made the time." But now that her child has grown up and left home, she wants to resume a more active sex life. This book can be of use, although Jim may need more direct assistance than he will get from Hilary reading this book and telling him about it.

The same holds true for Barbara. Barbara is a forty-nine-year-old physician who had her daughter when she was forty-two. Barbara says that she had no sex drive at all for about three years after her daughter was born. "And then, I think I was hit by some kind of hormone storm. Wow!" When Barbara's interest peaked, her husband had no interest at all. "He was chronically depressed and his depression and the meds affected his sex drive." So, Barbara thinks about old lovers and masturbates. "Besides this, he is a good husband and a good father, so I have no intention of leaving the relationship. Still, I wish it were different." Barbara and her husband would benefit from a self-help book geared for their situation, rather than for one aimed at low-desire women.

While Barbara's husband lost his drive due to his own personal issues, sometimes a husband's lost interest is due to his wife's repeated rebuffs to his sexual invitations. "I was too tired for so long that I always said no," says Jane. "Then, finally, once I approached him and he said no." Perhaps Jane's husband, Rob, was angry, hurt, or scared. Either way, according to Jane, "It wasn't a slippery slope. It was a dead end." Still, Jane feels that if she can open the conversation with Rob, it will be okay. If, like Jane, this is your situation, read on. If you think things have gone so far that you cannot talk to or work with your spouse to improve your sex life, then you may want to seek couples counseling instead. Or read on until the *Talk* step and give the suggested initial conversation a try. Depending on how it goes, you can decide if this book can help or if you need the assistance of a professional.

> *I was too tired for so long that I always said no. Then, finally, once I approached him and he said no.*
> —Jane, 52

### Our Stress Is Ripping Us Apart

Another couple's issue that can dampen desire is joint stress. Talking of the shared stress of dealing with their teen son's alcohol use, Allison says, "It's a constant struggle to be civil to each other much less wanting to touch." Allison could benefit from this book to help deal with her own stress, as well as to learn to better communicate with her husband about their shared stressors.

### We're Disconnected

A final issue of note is lack of connectedness. Sexual intimacy takes time to cultivate, even in couples that have been married a long time. In our busy lives, we often forget to spend time with our spouses and this inhibits sexual connection. If this issue is driving your diminished desire, this book is for you.

# Bad Loving

A reason that some women lose their sex drive is lack of good loving. While this is certainly a relationship issue, it is also worthy of its own focus. Mary and Wendy illustrate how bad loving can cause a woman's sex drive to plummet.

Wendy is a thirty-seven-year-old insurance agent. Until recently, she was satisfied with her sex life. Lately, her husband started watching a lot of hard-core pornography and wanting Wendy to do the things he saw in the movies. Although Wendy said no, he still changed his way of relating to her sexually. He was much more focused on his pleasure and less on pleasing her or getting her excited prior to intercourse. Intercourse became forceful and quick. Wendy and her husband need couples counseling, not this book.

The same is true for Mary. Mary is a forty-two-year-old mother of a teen boy who works as a secretary in a large law firm. She says that she could care less if she ever has sex again. When asked about sex, she tells the following story: "I was in the shower one morning, getting ready for work. Brent steps in with a big smile on his face. He gets behind me and starts to rub up against me and play with my boobs. He is getting all excited and says, 'Bend over baby.' I figured what the heck, and so I did and we had sex. He was thrilled and I figured that at least I got that chore over with for the week." Women certainly need a whole lot more caressing before intercourse than Mary got! While this is an extreme example, it illustrates the point that a husband's techniques can contribute to lack of interest in sex.

A husband not taking the time to arouse his wife in the way that gets her hot, throbbing, and wet can diminish interest in sex. Likewise, a husband's poor loving techniques can be at the root of a woman not having orgasms. A husband who doesn't know where his wife's clitoris is located is unlikely to have a wife who is going to desire sex with him or have orgasms. As will be emphasized in the *Touch* step, tired women need more caressing and foreplay than women who are not exhausted.

Are you exhausted and stressed? Do you know what kind of stimulation brings you the most excitement? Are you able to convey this to your husband? Does your husband take the time to pleasure you in a way that you find arousing? If you are wiped out and your husband doesn't take the time you need to get you excited, or you don't know how to tell him, this book is for you. If you are not tired but still have these other concerns, you can still benefit from this book; the *Talk* and *Touch* steps will help. You may also want to recommend that your husband read a book on pleasing women.

## Mistaking Other Sexual Problems for Low Desire

When Mary bent over in the shower, it is likely that she didn't lubricate before intercourse. She may have even experienced pain, due to the lack of foreplay before intercourse. She certainly didn't orgasm. All of this was due to her husband's lack of arousing her, as well as her not asserting her sexual needs. But, there are other cases where inability to orgasm, lack of lubrication, and pain during intercourse are independent sexual concerns. All of these can cause, or be confused with, diminished desire.

### Sexual Pain Problems

There are two types of sexual pain problems that women experience. One is when the muscles tighten up when the penis enters into the vagina. If you have lost your desire because this is happening to you, this book won't help. Skip to Appendix A and find a good sex therapist.

The other type of sexual pain occurs during intercourse. This kind of pain can range from mild to very intense. While it may be stating the obvious, if intercourse hurts, you won't want to engage in it. Pain during intercourse can be caused by lack of lubrication. It can also have medical or psychological causes. If you have lost your desire because intercourse hurts and you think this is because you aren't lubricating, read on. If you seem to be lubricating but still have pain during intercourse, rule out medical causes by seeing a well-informed and competent physician. It will be especially important to seek a physician experienced in treating vulvodynia, a medical condition that involves pain with penetration and can even produce pain when intercourse is not being attempted. If no medical causes or cures for the pain can be found, the next step would be to seek a knowledgeable sex therapist.

### Problems with Lubrication

If you aren't lubricating and feeling excited, you aren't going to want to have sex and your desire will decrease. Common but little-known causes of vaginal dryness include swimming pool chemicals, hot tub chemicals, harsh soaps and detergents, feminine douching products, overuse of caffeine and alcohol, cigarettes, lack of omega-3 fatty acids in one's diet, and dehydration. If you are suffering from vaginal dryness, experiment with these causes. For example, if you are douching, stop and see what happens. As another example, try adding more foods rich in omega-3 fatty acids to your diet.

Certain medications can cause vaginal dryness, including bladder and allergy medicines and some birth control pills. If you are taking medications and vaginal dryness is why you aren't in the mood, talk to your doctor to see if there are other medicines available.

Some medical issues diminish lubrication. Sexually transmitted infections (STIs) can lead to painful intercourse and lubrication problems years later. A host of current medical problems, such as diabetes, are associated with decreased lubrication. If you had an STI or have a medical issue, ask your doctor if this condition is associated with decreased lubrication. Likewise, vaginal dryness is a common symptoms associated with both breastfeeding and menopause.

There are many effective ways to treat vaginal dryness, including over-the-counter vaginal lubricants. Some are designed to be applied during sex (e.g., many K-Y brand products; Astroglide), whereas others (e.g., Replens) are designed as a longer-lasting (e.g., three-day) vaginal moisturizer. Some women find relief by squirting vitamin E oil in their vaginas. *Zestra* is a blend of botanicals available at most drug stores; one study found that when used as a genital massage oil, lubrication, desire, pleasure, and orgasm increased. For women for whom such over-the-counter remedies don't work, vaginally inserted estrogen creams, tablets, or slow-release rings are often prescribed. The North American Menopause Society recently concluded that women could stay on vaginal estrogen as long as needed, if other symptoms such as vaginal bleeding, spotting, and breast pain did not occur.

Marie, a fifty-three-year-old woman, received relief from an estrogen suppository. Marie was never in the mood and when she did have sex, it wasn't any fun because she was so dry. Upon examination, her physician saw that her vaginal walls were dry and prescribed an estrogen suppository. Marie began to lubricate again, both during sex and when thinking about sex. The sensation of lubrication got her in the mood again. Marie didn't need psychological help, she simply needed lubrication.

***meet jill,*** a fifty-one-year-old-woman who needed more than lubricants. Jill works about sixty hours a week as a manager of a small corporation, and is caring for aging parents. She has hot flashes during the day and night sweats that disturb her sleep. To cope with the vaginal dryness during the obligatory sex that she engages in, she experimented with a number of over-the-counter lubricants. While they helped with lubrication, Jill's sex drive remained at rock bottom. Jill's lost libido was due to both dryness *and* the stress of her life. She needed lubricants and the treatment offered here.

If the reason you are not interested in sex is vaginal dryness, try some of the over-the-counter-lubricants mentioned earlier. If they don't work, see your physician who may prescribe a cream, ring or suppository. If this does the trick, good for you! On the other hand, many of you will need lubricants plus the ideas presented in this book to deal with the other possible reasons for your dryness, including stress.

### Inability to Orgasm

Women who don't lubricate are less likely to orgasm. Nevertheless, problems with orgasm are an independent sexual issue that needs attention. Problems with orgasm are generally a lifelong issue. Once a woman learns how to reach orgasm, it is infrequent that she loses that capacity, except for when dealing with relationship turmoil, trauma, a medical condition, or a psychological issue. Also, some antidepressant medications inhibit women's orgasms. One study found that *Zestra*, the botanical oil mentioned above, increased arousal and orgasm even in women taking antidepressants. Another way to treat orgasm problems, as well as lubrication issues, that have a medical basis (such as diabetes or cervical irradiation) is with the FDA-approved Clitoral Therapy Device (EROS). The EROS provides gentle suction to the clitoris. This gentle suction increases blood flow to the area, which leads to clitoral engorgement. The EROS device is used intermittently during masturbation or foreplay, and studies report that it results in enhanced genital sensation, greater vaginal lubrication, improved ability to experience orgasm, and greater sexual satisfaction.

If your lack of interest in sex is because of problems with orgasm—lifelong or recently acquired due to trauma, a medical issue, or havoc in your relationship—this book isn't for you. Try a book designed to help women learn to orgasm, or seek medical or psychological help. If your lack of having an orgasm or lubricating might be stress-related, read on.

## Rushed Lifestyles and Hurried Sex: We're Back to Stress

A little-known, yet regular cause of vaginal dryness is stress. Stress is an especially common reason for vaginal dryness in women prior to perimenopause. As stated by Marcy Holmes, a nurse and writer for a website on women's health (*www.women towomen.com*), "After I hit thirty, I was working ten-hour days, getting very little sleep, stressed out, drinking too much coffee with not enough water intake, and not eating as well as I could. When I started experiencing vaginal dryness, I worried that I was in early menopause. But in looking back, I realized that I was pushing my body to the limit without enough support, and making little to no time for restorative behavior or sexual thinking." Related, when a woman tries to get sex over quickly so she can go to sleep, she isn't likely to lubricate or orgasm. This rushed sex further diminishes desire. Can you relate? If so, this book will offer you a six-step treatment program to reclaim desire. But, even before embarking on this program, a step you can take is to think of desire differently.

## Redefining Desire

Until now, you have been so focused on your missing physical desire that you may have failed to notice that you already have a psychological desire for sex. It's the reason you're reading this book. You already possess the wish to have sex regain its importance in your life. Now all we need to do is build upon this desire.

# Chapter 3

# Sex: Free, Fun, and Good For You!

Even if you have said "I don't care if I ever have sex again," a part of you doesn't mean this. You aren't indifferent to sex, or you wouldn't be reading this book. While you don't yet have the physical desire for sex, you already want sex to become a more central part of your life. This chapter aims to cement your psychological desire more firmly by getting you in touch with reasons to reclaim your sexual desire.

## A Rare Find

Sex feels good. When all is in balance in our lives, our bodies yearn for sex and react with ecstasy to sexual stimulation. As stated by Martha, a thirty-five-year-old client when describing her orgasms, "It's the most unique feeling in the world. Each one is different but no matter what, it's an amazing sensation." The #1 benefit of sex is that it feels wonderful.

This is only the tip of the iceberg. Sex is a rare find: it feels good, is good for you, and is free! In this chapter, the benefits of sex are categorized into physical health benefits, emotional health benefits, and relationship benefits. Some of the benefits are widely known and researched and others are more obscure, perhaps mentioned by only one study, physician, or psychologist. Several can be explained by hormones secreted during sex, including estrogen, testosterone, and oxytocin. While these biochemical causes are occasionally mentioned in this book, they aren't the focus of our discussion. The point is that sex is good for you!

Brian, a forty-year-old male client, recently told me that he has "great respect for the sex drive." He said sex is as vital to one's health as eating. Brian holds sex in high regard because he knows it is critical to his personal well-being and to his satisfaction with his marriage. If Brian lost his drive, he would fight to get it back. By the time you are done reading this chapter, I hope you are convinced you want to do the same. I hope you will more deeply realize that being too tired for sex is not a healthy choice and that it is time to reap the benefits of sex!

As you read about these perks, circle the ones that resonate with you. For example, if the deep sleep you used to fall into after sex is something you long to reclaim, circle this. Perhaps you never knew that sex might give you pain relief and given your frequent headaches, this appeals to you. If so, circle this.

## It's Great for Your Body

Although every woman may not derive every possible health benefit from sex, there are so many that you may as well reap the benefits of *some* of them!

*Sex is good exercise.* Intercourse is moderate exercise. It burns about 300 calories an hour, which equates to about five calories a minute. In addition, sex stretches and tones many muscles in your body. Intercourse may be especially helpful in toning your tummy, thighs, and buttocks.

*Sex is good for your posture.* This may be due to the workout your get from it or because you stand up taller when you feel good about yourself.

*Sex is good for your pain relief.* Sex can lower levels of pain associated with arthritis, whiplash, and headaches. Sex may relieve the tension that restricts the blood vessels that cause some headaches. Having an orgasm may be especially useful for pain relief; in one laboratory study conducted on real women, orgasm was found to increase a woman's pain threshold, as well as lessen her ability to detect pain.

*Sex is good for PMS.* One type of pain alleviated by sex is menstrual pain. Orgasm is especially effective in relieving PMS.

*Sex is good for your heart.* During arousal, your heart rate elevates. This is good for heart health.

*Sex is good for your vaginal health.* Women who orgasm frequently during their periods may have a lower risk of developing endometriosis than those who don't have frequent orgasms during their periods. Those who have more regular sexual contact with a partner may also have more regular periods. The blood flow to your vagina during sexual activity helps prevent vaginal dryness. The hormones secreted during sexual activity help keep your vaginal tissues smooth and supple. More than one physician and sex therapist has been quoted as saying that when it comes to vaginal health, it is a use-it-or-lose-it situation.

*Sex is good for your appearance.* In one study, a panel of judges viewed participants through a one-way mirror and guessed their ages. Those who looked seven- to twelve-years younger than their age were the women who were having the most sex. While some may argue this is because more attractive women have more sex, the evidence suggests that sex itself improves appearance. Sex improves overall health and generally, healthy people look better.

*Sex is good for your bladder.* Often, during intercourse, women flex their Kegel muscles, a group of muscles that support the bladder, urethra, and vagina. During orgasm, these same muscles involuntarily contract. Such muscle flexing and contracting improves bladder health and decreases your chance of having an incontinence-related problem.

*Sex is good for your digestive system.* Many women report that their digestive system works better after sex. This may be due to the exercise women get during sex, since regular exercise improves digestive health and relieves constipation. Sally laughingly refers to intercourse as her "best ever laxative." She almost always has a good bowel movement within a day after sexual intercourse.

*Sex is good for your immune system.* In one study, women who had genital contact or stimulation from their partner once or twice a week had higher amounts of immunoglobulin A (an antibody that is the body's first line of defense in fighting off disease and infections) than those who had sex less than once a week or not at all. Maybe this is why more frequent sex prevents colds and flu.

*Sex is good for your sense of smell.* In one study, albeit conducted with mice, mating increased olfactory sensitivity, including the ability to discriminate odors. Some hypothesize that sex has this same effect on humans. Perhaps this is why some people have positive odor memories or associations to sex, or why some people love the smell of sex. I have one friend, Olivia, who tells me that she can smell sex on herself for hours afterward. Olivia adores smelling the scent of sex on her body.

*Sex is good for your dental health.* Kissing is good for your teeth. Kissing produces saliva, which washes food away from teeth and lowers the level of the acid that causes decay. Also, since many people brush their teeth before sex, this promotes better dental hygiene. The more you have sex, the more brushing you do!

*Sex is good for your blood pressure.* Both sex and affectionate touch lower blood pressure. One study found that women who get daily hugs from their husbands have higher levels of the hormone oxytocin (often called the bonding hormone). Oxytocin lowers blood pressure. In fact, the decrease in blood pressure that daily hugging gives women is about the same as they might get from many blood pressure medications! Hugging isn't the only type of contact that lowers blood pressure. In one study, increases in blood pressure as a result of stress were less for those who had recently had intercourse than for those who hadn't.

*Sex is good for your cravings.* In two studies, one with mice and one with rats, the hormone oxytocin was related to consumption. In one of the studies, not having enough oxytocin was related to overeating. In the other, addicted rats given doses of oxytocin used less heroin. Perhaps this is why some women's cravings for food decrease after sex. Women often use food to console themselves, and after a lovely sexual or affectionate encounter, eating for comfort is not needed. Sex itself is the comfort.

## It Might Save His Life

Sex will contribute to your husband's health. One study found that men who have intercourse more often are less likely to develop erectile dysfunction. So, the more your husband uses his penis, the better it will work! Additionally, recent studies have found that men who ejaculate frequently may be protecting themselves against prostate cancer. Men's bones may also be made stronger by the increased testosterone secreted during sex. Finally, despite stories of men having heart attacks during sex, one study followed a group of forty-five to fifty-nine year-old men for twenty years and found that men who had intercourse two or more times a week cut their risk of having a fatal heart attack in half, when compared to men who had intercourse less than once a month. Looking at these same men across a ten-year time-span, mortality risk was 50% lower in men who reported a high frequency of orgasm when compared with men who reported a low frequency. So, botton line: by having intercourse with your husband, you will be improving his health—maybe even saving his life!

## A Mood Boost

Sex has some very potent emotional health benefits. Most of these benefits are more immediate and easily detectable than the physical health benefits. While you aren't likely to notice the dental health benefits of sex, the powerful stress relief you get is palpable. Nine sweeping emotional benefits are listed below. They all relate to you being more content.

*Sex enhances serenity.* One of the greatest ironies is that tired women are too stressed for sex, yet sex is one of the best stress relievers available. The stress relief benefits of sex are both immediately felt and enduring. While you are fully engaged in a sexual encounter, your mind is transported away from other worries. You can't be worrying about a problem at work and having an orgasm at the same time. In fact, one small neurological study found that as women were stimulated sexually, activity within the areas of the brain responsible for alertness and anxiety decreased. Strikingly, during orgasm, the area of the brain responsible for emotions, such as fear and anxiety, completely shut down. So, sex is an instant way to forget your woes and de-stress. Sex's stress relief benefits also linger on for hours and even days. The similarity between the slang expressions "well-laid" and "laid back" seems more than coincidental: a well-laid person feels laid back.

*Sex enhances patience.* Sex makes you less irritable. Annoyances are minimized and the things that bother you before sex often seem unimportant after sex.

*Sex enhances happiness.* After a satisfying sexual encounter, people report feelings of overall well-being, joy, and even euphoria. These feelings of happiness are enduring; studies find that the happier you are with your sex life, the happier you are in general. Your husband may be proud to learn that one study found that semen may have an antidepressant effect: women who regularly absorbed semen vaginally (through intercourse) or ingested it orally (through swallowing during oral sex) had decreased rates of depression.

*Sex enhances a zest for life.* When you let yourself immerse fully in the pleasure of sex, it can enliven you. Allowing yourself to be fully in touch with sexual pleasure can inspire you to appreciate and embrace all of life's pleasures.

*Sex enhances a positive outlook.* After good sex, the world looks like a brighter place. Laughter comes freer and easier after sex.

*Sex enhances a deeper connection with one's body and soul.* Sex helps get women out of their heads and into their bodies. Some women say sex enhances the spiritual aspect of their life. These women think of sexual energy as a spiritual force. They describe the experience of fully immersing in sexual pleasure and having an orgasm as a transcendent state that connects them with a core, spiritual part of themselves. Perhaps this benefit explains why some ancient, as well as modern, religions consider sex to be a sacred act.

*Sex enhances self-esteem.* The positive physical and emotional feelings associated with sex can make you feel good about yourself. Likewise, being sexually desired by your spouse and able to give him sexual pleasure can add to these positive feelings.

*Sex enhances self-care.* Having sex regularly seems to motivate women to attend to their other physical self-care needs, such as exercise and good nutrition. In the *Time* step, you will learn how self-care, such as exercise, can increase your sex drive. So, there is a positive cycle here: sex leads to self-care and self-care leads to sex.

*Sex enhances sleep.* The profound sense of emotional and physical peace following sex often leads one to fall into a deep and satisfying sleep. Recall that there is a vicious cycle occurring among many women. They try to jam too much into one day and the result is worry, which leads to restless sleep. Lack of sleep, in turn, is a real libido killer. An end to this vicious cycle is sex itself. A woman who crawls in bed exhausted but who can nevertheless muster the energy for sex is likely to sleep more soundly and more peacefully. She is also likely to awaken more rested and in a better mood the next morning. As stated by Nadine, a seventy-five-year-old woman who has had a satisfying sex life over the course of her fifty-five-year marriage, "During the most stressful times of my life, I liked sex the best. Even if I didn't have an orgasm, all that affection helped me fall into a really deep sleep. And, I would wake up feeling much better the next morning."

> *During the most stressful times of my life, I liked sex the best. ... All that affection helped me fall into a really deep sleep. .... I would wake up feeling much better the next morning.*
> —Nadine, 75

Undeniably, the emotional benefits of sex are all about mood enhancement. Certainly, if you and your husband are both in better moods, you will be happier together. This is just one of the many relationship benefits of sex, our next topic.

# Glue and Oil

Sex is the glue that holds marriage together. Without sex, marriages can fall apart or become only a partnership of shared chores and worries, with an occasional good laugh and conversation at best and much annoyance at each other at worst. As stated by Dianna, a woman you met in Chapter 2, "Marty and I have a lot of points of agreement and harmony. But, I can get that from my sister, my friends, and co-workers. I need more from my marriage." Dianna needs the glue of sex. And, honestly, Dianna can't just apply this adhesive once every blue moon and expect it to do its job. Sex is the kind of bonding agent that you need to keep re-applying. If you don't, your marriage is destined to be less happy at best and fall apart at worst.

Women and men in sexless relationships are prone to leave the relationship or to stay in the relationship but seek sex elsewhere.

In the nationally syndicated *On Ethics* column, Randy Cohen responded to a husband's disgruntled confusion about his wife saying that she didn't want to have sex anymore yet being angry he was having an affair. Randy Cohen said, "What your wife wants is not mere fidelity, of course, but the repudiation of what for many people is a profound and exultant part of life." Still, said Mr. Cohen, a dishonest affair is not the answer. He said that "She may not compel you to join her in forsaking sex but she may demand your honesty, regard, and considerations. Your desire is worthy of respect; your deceit is not." He advocated an honest discussion among this couple (and those like them) of their options, pointing out that one is for the couple to agree that the husband can seek sex elsewhere, if he does so in a way that doesn't cause his wife embarrassment. Certainly, this isn't the option you want or you wouldn't be reading this book. Still, Mr. Cohen's column is a to-the-point reminder that even though you have lost your drive, your spouse shouldn't be asked to give up what he considers a vital part of himself.

You need the relationship glue of sex to keep your marriage intact. But, sex is more than glue to hold your marriage rigidly together. At the same time, it is oil that keeps it running smoothly and prevents friction. Below are some of the more specific benefits of sex for your relationship and some of the essential reasons why you need to make your sex drive a priority in your life again.

*Sex creates intimacy.* Sex is the most intimate encounter two people can have. There is no distance between you and your husband during sexual intercourse; you are literally connected to one another in body and ideally, in soul. Sex enhances existing intimacy and helps you and your husband reach a new level of intimacy.

*Sex creates trust.* During sex, you and your husband are ideally sharing your most open and available selves with one another. Such vulnerability enhances trust.

*Sex creates shared memories.* You and your husband are creating special, shared memories when you have sex. You can put these memories to use later: many couples find sexual reminiscing together to be an effective way to rekindle the mood.

*Sex creates shared secrets with your spouse.* After sex, couples exude the feeling that they have a special shared secret. Couples often develop special words to refer to sex. Couples also often share laughter and jokes during sex—jokes that become a special, shared part of their relationship. My clients Lisa and Alex refer to sex as making a spaghetti dinner and so have a language that only they share ("Do you want to have spaghetti tonight?").

*Sex creates a stronger commitment.* Couples that have a good sexual relationship seem to be more deeply committed to one another. Also, generally, the better the sexual relationship in the marriage, the less likely either partner is going to look for it outside the relationship.

*Sex creates a deeper appreciation for one another.* Couples tend to notice the positive aspects of their partner's personality more after sex. Sex also raises our tolerance: things that one finds annoying before a sexual encounter are often not so annoying afterwards, or can even be endearing. Couples are definitely less snippy with each other after sex.

*Sex creates generosity in your relationship.* There may be some truth to the jokes about a woman having sex with her husband as a way to get him to agree to an expensive purchase. Research suggests that the hormones secreted during sex increase feelings of generosity. Regardless of the underlying reason, it does seem that you and your husband will be more giving after sex.

*Sex creates an opportunity for playfulness.* Sex can be intense and serious, but it can also be playful. Couples also seem more playful and lighthearted with one another after a sexual encounter.

*Sex creates a unique way to communicate love.* Sex is a one-of-a-kind way to communicate loving feelings. My client, Andrea, a fifty-eight-year-old woman, refers to sex with her husband as "talking with our bodies."

*Sex is the way that we talk with our bodies.*
—Andrea, 58

*Sex creates an opportunity to cuddle.* There is a lot of body contact before, during and after sex. Many women say that after-sex cuddling is the best.

*Sex creates more sex.* The more sex you have, the more you want. After a good sexual encounter, many a woman has said something along the lines of "I forgot how fun that is. We need to do that more often." Sex itself is the best medicine for your diminished desire! Finally, having sex does wonders to end the tension in a relationship over when sex is going to occur.

> *I forgot how fun that is.*
> *We need to do that more often!*
> —Countless women who say they
> are too tired for sex.

In short, sex is critical for marital health. The majority of therapists will tell you that it is actually necessary for a good marriage. While some couples will say that they don't have sex but are still happy together, they are often not facing their problem directly or are in denial about the toll that lack of sex is taking on their relationship.

Jim and Sally came to me for counseling concerning problems in their marriage, including a lack of sex. At first, they said that they wanted to have sex again but it wasn't necessary; they were happy without it. However, a year later when they were having regular sex, they expressed that they really hadn't been as happy together without sex as they first said. They were simply too scared to admit it.

A marriage that is suffering is also going to produce children that are less happy and emotionally well-adjusted. One of the strongest predictors of a child's adjustment is the strength of their parent's marital bond. Thus, if you have children, reviving your sex life is also going to benefit their well-being.

To recap, a sexual relationship creates good feelings between you and your spouse. As aptly stated by my fifty-two year old friend Teresa, a woman who has never lost her sex drive, "That is why they call it making love. It creates more love each time."

> *That's why they call it making love.*
> *It creates more love each time.*
> —Teresa, 52

## A Positive Cycle

While the benefits of sex were presented above in distinct categories (e.g., health, relationship), they are interconnected. A good sexual relationship is going to make you and your spouse happier, and research shows that happier people are physically healthier. Research shows that women in happier marriages have a lower risk of medical problems, ranging from the flu to cardiovascular problems, than women in stressful marriages. Being happier as a result of a good sexual relationship will also lead you and your husband to be more open to one another. You will be more affectionate, more trusting, and more caring. You will show more interest in one another and be more giving to one another. You will notice the good in one another more intensely and be much less critical and snippy about the minor annoyances. You will do things for one another more freely. The love will sparkle in your eyes again as you look at one another. You will feel loved and cared about, and will touch each other affectionately more often. All this will lead you to feel better about yourself and your marriage. In short, sex sparks a wonderful circle of benefits: Enhanced physical health, a happier relationship, more sex—and the cycle goes on.

## Your Inspiration for Sex

Hopefully, you now see all the amazing benefits of sex! Now it is time to zero in on the most important reasons that you want to reclaim your desire.

If you circled reasons as you read, take a moment and look over what you circled. Then, put a star next to your top reason to reclaim your desire. If you didn't circle as you read, take a moment to skim the reasons and star the one that stands out to you. However, if too many of these reasons look good to you, you can simply think about the general principles in this chapter as reasons to reclaim your desire. These principles are:

- *Sex feels wonderful.*
- *Sex is good for your physical health.*
- *Sex enhances your emotional health.*
- *Sex creates a loving, trusting, committed relationship.*

Circle the one that appeals to you most. Or, if you can't narrow it down even this much, perhaps you have simply realized that sex is both fun and good for you! Sex is medicine for your body, your soul, and your relationship! Indeed, sex itself is the cure for your waning libido. The first step you can take is to start thinking about sex again; this comes in the next chapter.

*Chapter 4*

# The Sex Organ above Your Neck: Thoughts for Tired Women

*It starts in your head. If your head isn't there, the mechanics don't matter.*

—Jean, 49

Your most important sex organ is located between your ears. I once told a client this and she countered with "Wow! All these years, I thought it was someplace else!" She was referring to her clitoris, the orgasm hot button. But, as stated by Jean, "It starts in your head. If your head isn't there, the mechanics don't matter." What Jean was saying is that all the clitoral stimulation in the world isn't going to do much good if the woman receiving it is writing her to-do list in her head, or as Sandra once reported to me, calculating the number of hours of sleep she would get and worrying about how tired she would be the next day. This type of mindset is not going to enhance sexual desire or pleasure!

To enjoy sex, you must develop the proper state of mind. To reclaim your sexual desire, you will need to focus on it, both throughout the day and during sexual encounters. Your thoughts are of critical importance, both in general and about sex in particular.

## Thoughts: The Gateway to Change

Cognitive therapy helps people to change their thought patterns and is one of the most effective forms of treatment that exists for a multitude of problems. Cognitive therapy is based on the idea that it is not events that influence our emotions but our thoughts about these events that are key. Some of our thoughts are within our conscious awareness (we know we are thinking them) and some are unconscious (we think them automatically without awareness). Cognitive therapy helps people to identify both types of negative thoughts and to substitute these downbeat thoughts with more positive ones. While this sounds simple, changing thoughts requires focused effort and practice. Even though as a psychologist I am well-versed in the power of positive thinking, it is not something that comes naturally to me. Allow me to illustrate with two examples, one in which my thinking is obvious to me and one in which it is more automatic.

My house is less tidy than I would prefer. There are often baskets of clean but unfolded laundry in my living room and piles of other family member's belongings scattered throughout the house. How much this bothers me is dependent on how I think about the mess. When I allow myself to think, "This house is such a mess! I hate it!" then I feel and act cranky. However, if instead, I can remember to take a deep breath and think, "My house looks like a relaxed and loving place for my family" or "I will miss the mess when the girls leave home" then the disarray truly doesn't bother me. The clutter hasn't changed, only my attitude about it has changed. This attitude shift results in me feeling more positively in my home.

The same applies to how I react when my daughters interrupt me when I am working from home. Although I often work from home specifically so I can be available for my children, when they interrupt me I sometimes experience an instantaneous flash of irritability. When this happens, I use my irritation as a cue that my thoughts need to change. As soon as I feel my edginess, and ideally before I express it, I take a deep breath and think something positive and calming such as "I am so lucky to be here for my children" or "Enjoy the time helping them." My irritation instantly fades, and this is because I have changed my thinking. I substituted a thought that came so fast that I wasn't even aware of it ("I can never get anything done!") to one that is more constructive. In doing so, my emotions become more positive.

Both of these examples illustrate the central principle of cognitive therapy: changing negative thoughts to positive ones is the gateway to change. The first step to getting your desire back is the way you think about it. Reclaiming passion starts with the belief that you need to reclaim it and that you want to reclaim it. Before again feeling spontaneous vaginal lubrication, you must first grease the wheels of your mind.

## Daily Foreplay for Your Mind

The notion that every day is foreplay is one you will see reflected throughout this book. We generally think of foreplay as the caressing and touching that occurs before intercourse, but it is more useful to think of foreplay in a much broader way. Foreplay is all that you do to get yourself interested in and ready for sex. The first act of foreplay happens in that vital sex organ between your ears: your brain.

Several thought-related foreplay techniques are described below. While changing thoughts sounds simple, doing so takes effort. Akin to a physical exercise program, it's easy to start with enthusiasm and then slowly stop the routine. If this happens, just keep starting over until the process becomes part of your daily routine.

### See Sex Everywhere

I have two friends who enjoy a vibrant sex life. One never lost her sex drive and the other did and has regained it—with full force! What these women have in common is that they both think about sex a lot, despite balancing high-pressure jobs, children, and the many demands of life.

Teresa is a fifty-two-year-old teacher and the mother of a junior in college. She tries to notice the sexual and the sensual in all that she does and all that surrounds her. She wears clothes that feel sensual to her skin. She notices other people flirting with each other. Teresa savors flavors that she likes, eating the food slowly and purposefully. She takes the time to stop and smell things that she likes, including flowers as we walk and vanilla as she cooks. She often burns candles or incense. Teresa is in touch with all of her senses and allows herself to enjoy the pleasure of each fully. Such a focus clearly enhances her sexuality. Teresa consistently sees and purposefully focuses on sexuality and sensuality in the world around her, and credits this as the reason her sex drive has stayed consistently high.

Amy is an engineer who has two children, one of whom has a physical disability. For years, she was so exhausted that she had no sex drive. When I asked Amy how she regained her sex drive, she told me that she simply started thinking about and focusing on sex. We were at a professional lunch at the time and she told me that right that very moment, she was undressing various men in her mind and imagining what they would be like in bed. Amy pointed to a rather attractive man in the room and whispered in my ear about all the things she was fantasizing doing with him. She told me that she does this a lot during professional meetings. Amy explained that this makes meetings less boring, and builds up sexual energy that she takes home to her husband at night.

## thought *homework*

Notice and focus on both sensuality and sexuality. Focus fully and intensely on all five of your senses: touch, sight, hearing, smell, and taste. Observe and take in the sexual energy exuded by the people around you. Revel in this energy.

## Fantasize Daily

Closely related to seeing sexuality all around you is fantasizing about sex. As you can see from reading about Amy, who covertly undresses men in professional meetings, there is only a small step between thinking about sex and imagining sexual scenes. Amy also fantasizes about imaginary or past sexual scenes. She also flexes her Kegel muscles as she fantasizes, or in other words, she squeezes and releases the muscles in her vagina and pelvis.

"Fantasy and Kegel exercises go together like popcorn and a movie," she declares.

Focusing your thoughts and imagery on sex is critical to regaining your sex drive. You are stressed and preoccupied and because of this, thoughts about sex are rarely going to bubble up spontaneously. You thus need to consciously focus your thoughts and images on sexual scenes. Teresa, the woman described earlier who has never lost her sex drive, intentionally works on this by "thinking and fantasizing every day how nice it feels to make love." Purposefully focusing on sexual thoughts and fantasies can help you recapture that deliciously aroused feeling you are trying to reclaim.

Even if you can barely recall what it feels like to be in the mood, you are reading this book because at one point you adored this feeling and the sex that it led you to seek out. You can use your past to get your thoughts going again. Likewise, you can use fantasy images—things that have never occurred in your life but that sound exciting to you.

> *Fantasy and Kegel exercises go together like popcorn and a movie.*
> —Amy, 38

Before prescribing your next assignment, however, let me issue a word of reassurance. Fantasies are different from reality. Many women feel guilty about their thoughts and thus don't use them to their advantage. I tell clients and my children that their thoughts are okay no matter what they are, and that they are different from actions. I tell my children that it is normal and acceptable to think negative thoughts about me ("My mom is so annoying!"), but it is not acceptable to speak disrespectfully to me. As it applies to the current exercise, there is no need to censor or judge your images, even if they aren't of your husband or seem bizarre or unusual. These images are ones that you don't ever need to share with anyone or act on. In allowing your mind total freedom you can recall an exciting past sexual encounter or create sexually stimulating fantasy images. You can then take the energy derived and use it in bed with your husband. Enjoy your thoughts without guilt!

### thought *homework*

Take a five-minute "sex break" in your mind once daily. Stop what you are doing and recall a peak sexual encounter from your past, such as one in which you had an amazing orgasm or one that was a bit unusual or especially exciting in terms of location. Another option for your five-minute sex break is to engage in a fantasy that is sexually titillating for you, even if it is something you would never actually do. Imagine, for example, an encounter with a sexy stranger that you just met. If you find it enhances your drive further, do your Kegel exercises as you fantasize. (This is when you squeeze and release muscles in your vagina; to find these muscles, try stopping and starting your flow of urine.)

### Find and Repeat Your Mantra

When working with clients, I often help them to develop a "mantra" that they repeat several times a day. Mantras work best when they are concise and tailor-made to fit the person's situation. To illustrate with a nonsexual example, Jason was working on getting tenure at a major research university and struggling with feeling inept. After brainstorming several options, we came up with the mantra of "I am a competent scientist." Jason repeated this mantra to himself several times a day, and the worries and fear slowly dissipated.

A more sexually focused example involves Amber, the woman whose decreased desire stemmed from thoughts about her husband feeling like her brother. The core problem for Amber was the belief that as emotional intimacy increases, sexual excitement decreases. To turn this around, Amber needed to delete this detrimental thought from her subconscious and replace it with a new, more productive thought. Amber's mantra was "Emotional closeness turns me on." This mantra helped Amber overcome her damaging belief that sex was best reserved for those we aren't close with.

The effectiveness of a personal mantra lies in the principles of cognitive therapy outlined earlier, as well in repetitive practice. Mantras work by replacing negative thoughts with positive ones, and by focusing you intentionally on the positive thoughts.

### ERASE THESE THOUGHTS

Below are some things that you may think about sex, either consciously or unconsciously.

- *I'm too tired for sex.*
- *I'm too busy for sex.*
- *I have no interest in sex.*
- *I don't care if I ever have sex again.*
- *I don't enjoy sex anymore.*
- *Sex is one more chore on my to-do list.*

- *Sex is something I do for my husband.*
- *I would much rather read or watch television than have sex.*
- *Sex takes too much energy at the end of a long day.*
- *All the hours I have in bed I need for sleeping.*

Do these resonate with you? What other negative thoughts about sex have you had?

Now it is time to ERASE these negative thoughts and replace them with more positive thoughts.

## JOYFUL THOUGHTS OF SEX

Below are the same negative thoughts listed above turned into positive ones:

- *Sex revitalizes me!*
- *I'm never too busy for sex!*
- *I love sex!*
- *I'm going to have great sex!*
- *I am passionate!*
- *Sex is my reward!*
- *Sex is what I do for me!*
- *I'd rather have sex than anything else!*
- *Sex is my end of the day treat!*
- *Sex helps me sleep soundly!*

## YOUR PERSONAL MANTRA

Do any of these thoughts speak to you as the way that you would like to think? If so, use it as your mantra. If none of these thoughts work for you, let's develop one that does. Look back at the list of reasons for having sex in Chapter 3. Pick one that you circled as being important to you and turn that into a mantra. If you circled "Sex enhances feelings of closeness," you may want to think "Sex connects me with my husband." If you circled "Sex enhances laughter," you may want to think "Sex is good for my humor!" If "Sex enhances serenity" got your attention, experiment with "Sex calms me" or "I want to be well-laid and laid-back." Try out a few mantras, and let yourself see how they feel. Then, settle on one or two that fit best.

### thought *homework*

Say your mantra to yourself four times a day. Say this mantra to yourself before you get out of bed, twice during the day and as you get into bed at night.

### Seven Days of Foreplay

You will notice I just gave you three exercises, all involving foreplay of the mind. If you were my client, we would discuss which of these three you feel would work best for you. We would discuss if you wanted to try one of them, two of them, or all three of them. While I would encourage you to try all three strategies, I would also tell you to use your judgment about what was working and to make adjustments during the week. I would emphasize that the important thing was that you do something to get your daily thoughts focused on sex. Our session would end there and I would ask you to come back in a week and let me know how it went.

Hopefully, you would come back with good results to report. If so, I would urge you to keep this exercise going and remind you that thinking positively about sex needs to be a permanent change. On the other hand, if you came back with no change, we would readjust. We would develop a new mantra or examine your guilt about your fantasies, with me reassuring you that whatever you think is okay. Of course, I can't do this with you in a book format, so I ask you to do this for yourself. Try these strategies for a week and then come back and evaluate. Remember, though, that not every strategy will work for every woman.

Eve, a stay-at-home mother with two children, found that changing her thoughts was only effective to a point. Specifically, thoughts she thinks at 2:00 P.M. get her horny and she wishes she could act on them at that time. But, by the time she gets into bed at 10:00 P.M., the horniness has dissipated and sleep is her priority. Eve found the *Time* and *Tryst* strategies most helpful to recovering her drive. While the strategies in this book build upon one another, not every woman is going to get the same effects from each exercise. Still, read and try them all and you will find the ones that turn your drive back on again. The next strategy—focusing on sex during sex—is one that many women derive great benefit from.

## Mind-Blowing Sex: Focusing on Sex During Sex

Sandra tells me that about one in four times that she has sex, she has an orgasm. According to Sandra, this has more to do with her state of mind than with what her husband does. Her husband does the same things each time, and these are things that she likes very much. Still, how much she enjoys sex has to do with whether or not she allows herself to relax. In Sandra's words, "If I can't turn off my to-do list, then it's service-type sex. It isn't aversive—but it isn't great either. But, if I can relax and shut off my mind, then the sex can be awesome." Her sexual enjoyment depends on if she can turn off her mental to-do list and instead focus on the pleasure of the moment.

> *If I can't turn off my to-do list, then it's service-type sex. . . . But, if I can relax and shut off my mind, then the sex can be awesome.*
> —Sandra, 51

Does this sound familiar? It probably does, because mental chatter during sex is a common problem among women. Research shows that women get distracted more during sex than men do. Recently, a client told me that in the midst of an enjoyable sexual encounter, she noticed a mess in the bathroom that her husband had left when he was wallpapering. She reported experiencing an instantaneous diversion from the positive sexual feelings. She quickly went from feeling sexually aroused to feeling annoyed and unable to concentrate on the sex.

Women's distracting thoughts during sex usually have to do with parts of their bodies they don't like, things on their to-do list, or leftover issues from a busy day. Such mental multitasking during sex contributes to diminished desire. After all, who wants to have sex when it is just another time to think about all your worries? Also, thinking about tasks you have to do at a time that you can't do them is only going to increase your anxiety. And, anxiety is a real turn-off. You can't feel fretful and sexually aroused at the same time. Below are two strategies to help you focus on sex during sex.

## Channel Changing: From Mind to Body

If during sex you find your mind wandering to anything but the feelings and sensations in your body, you need to purposefully and intentionally stop these thoughts. You can think "Stop" to yourself. Or, you may want to try something gentler such as "Focus" or "Center." One of my clients cleverly came up with "Bed not Head." Some women report that looking deeply into their husband's eyes helps them to refocus. Touching a part of your husband's body that you find particularly appealing, such as his shoulders or cheek, can also be used to signal yourself to refocus during sex. Zeroing in with complete focus on wherever his hands are touching can help bring you back into the flow of the moment and its sensations. Breathing your husband's scent deeply can remind you to come back to the moment. Some women speak out loud to bring themselves into the present, giving their husbands instructions on how to touch them or engaging in dirty talk. These women say they can't be talking about sex and thinking about something else at the same time. The key is to find the refocusing signal that works best for you. Whichever signal you use, the principle is the same: when your mind wanders during sex, you need to firmly but gently signal yourself to change the channel in your mind.

Your next natural question is likely, "What channel should I change to?" The channel you want to change to is the one where you lose yourself in the physical sensations of the moment. The goal is to change the channel from your mind to your body, from your thoughts to your sensations. One client of mine, Kerry, reports that she tells herself to "breathe into your genitals." She then automatically breathes deeply and gets into what she calls "meditation mode." This is the same client who became distracted by the wallpaper mess in the bathroom, and she was able to use this method to refocus on the sex. Another client simply brings all of her energy to whatever body part her husband is touching. No matter how you get there, the goal is to have mindful sex.

## Mindful Sex

Giving one's complete attention to what is happening in the moment has garnered a great deal of attention among psychologists in recent years, although it has been part of Buddhist teachings for centuries. In a nutshell, mindfulness entails focusing completely and totally on what is happening in the present moment. I think of mindfulness as akin to riding a roller coaster. If you have ever been on a roller coaster—and whether you liked the experience or not—I bet you were thinking of nothing else but what was occurring that very moment. You were too immersed in flying downhill to think about the pile of work left at home or in the office.

In daily life, however, thoughts about one thing occur in the middle of doing other things. You think about a conversation with your boss in the middle of talking to your spouse. An e-mail you have to respond to pops into your head in the middle of making love with your husband. In mindfulness practice, distracting thoughts are noticed and observed and then released without judgment. In some forms of mindfulness practice, one is instructed to watch invasive thoughts float away or to imagine them being taken away on a conveyer belt. When practicing mindfulness, the key is to focus one's totality on what is happening in the present moment. We can be mindful during any activity. Washing the dishes, for example, can be a meditative, present moment if you completely immerse yourself in the feel of warm, sudsy water on your hands. Eating mindfully can enhance the pleasure of a meal. A state of total immersion and present-focus can be invoked during vacuuming, showering, or talking with a friend.

Practice mindfulness in all you do throughout the day. The more practiced you are at achieving an in-the-moment state, the easier it will be for you to achieve this same state during sex. Mindful sex is sex in which you are totally and completely immersed in the physical sensations of your body. The next time you have sex, have mindful sex. Allow yourself to indulge fully and completely in the physical sensations of the moment. If distracting thoughts occur, take a deep breath and let them float by without judgment. Allow your breaths to lead you fully back to your body's ecstatic physical reactions. Focus on being completely immersed in the sexual sensations.

***meet lydia,*** a fifty-one-year-old woman who recently used channel changing and a mindful focus to have awesome sex. It was a Saturday, and all three of her teenagers were out of the house. Although Lydia was stressed about work, she was aware that she and her husband hadn't had sex in a while. She talked to herself, reminding herself that she would feel less uptight after sex, as well as closer to her husband. So, even though she wasn't in the mood, she invited her husband to have sex with her and he readily agreed. For the first several minutes, thoughts of work kept popping in Lydia's head. She was distracted and not fully present, and so not lubricating sufficiently. But, she persisted, telling herself to "focus" and "breathe." When this didn't work, she recalled the notion of sex as something that takes women out of their head and into their bodies and souls. She told herself, "Allow this spiritual experience." This thought helped her direct her total attention on the sensations in her body, especially on her genitals as her husband caressed her clitoris. She ended up in a totally immersed state. She had a mind-blowing orgasm, the effects of which lasted throughout her more relaxed and peaceful day.

It is no coincidence that the phrase "mind-blowing" is often associated with sex. To reach mind-blowing sex, you have to engage in mindful sex. To have sensational sex, you have to focus on the sensations and not on your unwashed laundry or unfinished work project. Mind-blowing sex means that your mind is not working; only your body is reacting. Busy brains are not for the bedroom.

In the next chapter, you will learn to talk with your partner about what you need to help turn off your busy brain. But, your own thought processes—over which you have sole and total control—are the first step. Please remember this and keep working on the exercises in this chapter.

## Thought Step Wrap-Up

Your most important sex organ can be found between your ears, and using this sex organ wisely is going to help you recover your sex drive! To begin to get the most pleasure out of this sex organ as you can, use the three thought-related foreplay techniques for a week (see sex everywhere; fantasize daily; repeat your mantra). As you do, make adjustments to suit your needs, with the goal being to make having sexual thoughts become a lifestyle habit. Also, practice a mindful focus throughout the day during nonsexual activities to help you get there during sex. If you feel distracted during sex, change the channel from your brain to your bodily sensations. Have mindful sex by focusing completely on your in-the-moment physical sensations. In short, keep thinking sexy thoughts when you are not in bed and keep focusing on the sexual feelings when you are in bed!

*Chapter 5*

# "Oral" Sex: Talk for Tired Women

Hopefully, you are now thinking about sex. That is a private activity. Now it is time for a shared activity: Talk. It is time to focus on talking with your spouse and making improving your sex drive a matter that is between you and him.

## The "Bed Rock" of Intimacy

Take a moment to think about a female friend or relative that you feel close to. My guess is you thought of a person you like to talk with. Perhaps she listens well to your problems, makes you laugh, or gives you good advice. You thought of this friend because the way you and she communicate enhances your connection. As humans, we are bound together by our ability to communicate. Communication is central to our individual well-being and to our relationship satisfaction.

As a therapist, I have seen marriages ripped apart by poor communication and pieced back together again by good communication. In counseling couples, I often find that at the root of years of built-up pain and dissatisfaction is simply a lack of communication skills. Likewise, couples can't heal their rifts without talking and listening well to each other. The research backs up my observation: good communication is highly related to satisfaction in marriage. Quite pertinent, one study found that husbands and wives who talked more to one another were more sexually active. Communication is the bedrock of a good marriage, and good communication can help make your bed rock!

That is why one of my first steps when counseling couples, about sex or any other issue, is to teach them the principles and strategies of effective communication. The same holds true in individual counseling. In almost twenty years of counseling, I can't think of a client I've worked with whose communication style has not either contributed to their problems, been part of their recovery, or both. Most people in our culture have never been explicitly taught useful communication skills and those who have often forgo such skills when tight on time, exhausted, or upset. The ability to communicate effectively, particularly when hurt or angry, is an uncommon skill, but the key to relationship intimacy.

In this chapter, you will find information on general communication principles and skills that is not always tied to sexuality. This is because these communication principles and skills are foundational. As you read some sections below, don't be alarmed if sex isn't mentioned for several pages at a time. To get your sex drive back, we must first focus on the basic issue of effective communication. But, you alone learning effective general and sexual communication skills may or may not result in your relationship improving. Even when you learn new communication skills, positive responses from others are not guaranteed, especially if the other person doesn't know how to communicate effectively. To address this problem, the last section of this chapter focuses on bringing your husband on board. This section will center on talking with your husband about your quest to find your lost libido, how he can help, and new ways of talking with each other. This assumes that your husband is willing. Alicia described her husband as uncommunicative. She says, "He isn't a talker and sex was our link. It was the greatest body language in the world, and now without that, it's just empty space." Still, she predicted, once he understood that the outcome of talking would be sex, he would be more willing to talk. She was right. Like Alicia, you will be guided to talk with your husband at the end of this chapter and subsequent chapters will build on this.

## From Faulty Beliefs to Guiding Principles

Communication consists of both principles and skills. Principles are the things we believe to be true that guide our behaviors. Faulty beliefs about communication can be at the root of a couple's problems, either sexually or in general. Below are four faulty ways of thinking that erode relationships, as well as ways to flip such thinking around for enhanced marital connection and harmony. Indeed, when turned around, these four faulty beliefs become the four guiding principles of effective communication.

### I Shouldn't Have to Ask

Oftentimes during a counseling session with a couple, one of the partners will hint at something that they want from the other. I will then make this wish explicit by saying for example, "Janice, it sounds to me like you want Sam to spend more time with the kids on weekends." "Well yes, of course!" is the general reply I get after such a reflection. I then ask, "Have you told Sam this?" About half the time, the answer to such a question is "I shouldn't have to ask. He should know this!" This response is based on the mistaken belief that our partners should know what we want without us telling them.

No one can read minds, nor should they be expected to try. The attitude that people, particularly your spouse, should know what you want without you having to tell them is a sure-fire way to communicate ineffectively. To resent something that your partner is not giving you that you haven't clearly asked for is also groundless. Likewise, to be angry at someone for doing something you find distasteful but that you haven't told him is offensive is equally as unfounded. To have any chance of getting what you want, you have to learn to ask for it clearly. People, particularly spouses, can't be expected to guess our needs. We have to tell them.

Perhaps you're thinking that if you actually have to ask for something, then it is less meaningful to receive it. Instead of thinking that asking diminishes receiving, ponder instead how magnificent it can be to directly ask for something important to you and then receive it. This means that your partner listened to you and demonstrated his caring for you by giving you what you asked for. Of course, we can't always get what we ask for, but the only way to have a shot at getting it is to ask for it. Expecting our partners to mind-read is akin to expecting them to know what childbirth or menstruation feels like. They can't.

Perhaps right about now you are thinking that men are flawed because they can't mind-read, yet you and other women you know seem to be able to do so. Research shows that women are better at reading nonverbal cues than men are. Some speculate that this is due to women needing to read the nonverbal cues of infants more than men do. This ability to read nonverbal cues is likely at the root of what we call "women's intuition." Still, though, you can be totally wrong in your reading of nonverbal cues; your intuition can easily be off-base. Just as you cannot expect your spouse to read your mind, don't expect to be able to read his.

### I'm Sure I Know

Assuming that you know something can be hazardous to your marriage and to your sex life. You must check out your assumptions. To illustrate the power of checking out assumptions, let's take a couple in their mid-sixties who came to me for counseling.

**meet alex and lisa.** Alex was raised to believe that women don't like sex, and that it is something that they do grudgingly to keep men happy. Over the years, when he and Lisa would have sex, he would try to complete the sexual act as quickly as possible. He said he did this to be considerate of Lisa. He didn't want her to have to do something she didn't like for too long. In therapy, Alex had the opportunity to check out his assumption. At my urging, he asked Lisa, "Do you like sex?" He was very surprised to hear that she did. Getting rid of this false assumption opened the door for an explicit discussion about what Lisa and Alex each liked sexually. Each of them spent time telling the other directly and clearly what they wanted sexually. Perhaps not surprising to you, Lisa wanted Alex to take more time and engage in more touching of her before intercourse. He was eager to oblige, and the result is a newfound sexual satisfaction with each other, after almost thirty years of marriage!

### It's Useless to Discuss

Along with their sexual problems, Lisa and Alex had a host of other built up resentments. Thirty years of ineffective communication had led to a litany of things they each felt angry about. This is typical of couples that come to therapy and is why I tell my backpack story.

We all walk around with an invisible backpack on our backs for each significant relationship we are in. When things bother or upset us, we often don't tell each other. We may think it isn't worth it or we won't be able to solve the problem anyway. Each upset that we don't discuss is akin to a pebble. We walk along picking up pebble after pebble and putting them in our backpacks. Eventually the pebbles add up and the backpack is so heavy that it hurts to carry it. We dump it out, in an attempt to lighten our load. We start throwing the stones at each other.

My therapy with couples is focused on emptying the backpack and helping them to learn not to put pebbles in anymore. Couples need to get rid of the old stones by talking them through or by throwing them out, realizing that they were put into the backpack due to lack of communication. They have to learn the communication skills so that in the future, they don't hold onto pebbles.

## Winners and Losers

In our culture, we are often encouraged to argue to prove our point. We are taught to fight to win. This is rarely constructive and can lead to harm being done to the marital relationship. Instead, couples need to take the attitude that the purpose of disagreements is to get closer rather than to win. When in conflict with your spouse, the ideal goal is to resolve the issue sufficiently (even if that resolution is agreeing to disagree) so that you don't have to argue about it ever again. When you disagree, look at it as an opportunity to understand your spouse's viewpoint, to express yours, and grow closer in the process. It will be especially helpful if instead of getting defensive when your spouse is upset with you, you actually try to understand why they feel as they do.

### Four Guiding Principles

You just read about four faulty beliefs about communication that can erode relationships. You also heard about healthier attitudes about communication. Now, let's make these positive beliefs even more explicit. The four guiding principles of effective communication are:

1. Principle #1: Ask for what you want. Don't expect your spouse to mind-read.
2. Principle #2: Check out your assumptions.
3. Principle #3: Work out issues as they arise, rather than hold onto them in your metaphorical backpack.
4. Principle #4: Work to resolve issues rather than to win a fight.

## Eight Superb Communication Skills

Entire books have been written on communication skills. The eight skills below are those I find create the most positive change in couples' general and sexual relationships.

### Skill #1: Match What You Say with How You Say It

Communication skills consist of verbal components (what we say) and nonverbal components (the looks on our faces, our body posture). The nonverbal component is especially powerful. If your spouse or teenager was making a lot of noise while in the kitchen (slamming cabinet doors, banging pots and pans) but when you asked if they were mad, they said, "No, I'm not mad," you would likely still think they were mad. If you told your friend that you were interested in hearing about her problem but then kept glancing at your watch while she was talking, she would conclude that you were not really interested. When you say you are enjoying sex but are stifling yawns, your husband will decide that you aren't really into having sex. When verbal and nonverbal behaviors conflict, we assume that the nonverbal behaviors are the truthful ones.

Often women's nonverbal and verbal communication don't match because they're reluctant to say what they are feeling or wanting, or because they don't have the skills to do so. This chapter will help you match your verbal and nonverbal communications by providing you with the belief that you have the right to express your wants and by teaching you the skills to do so. It will also help you effectively confront your spouse when his verbal and nonverbal messages don't match. If your spouse asks if you want to have sex and you say you are too tired and he says this is fine, but then pouts, you can point this out. "I hear you say that you are fine with us not having sex, but I notice you are pouting. I would like to talk about this."

Sound unrealistic or hard to do? Read on for seven skills that will help you convey your needs and react appropriately to the needs of your spouse.

## Skill #2: Don't Ask Questions That Aren't Questions

Many people ask questions that aren't really questions at all. Both women and men do this, although women seem to do it more often. Asking a question that isn't a question is often something that people do, consciously or unconsciously, to avoid owning their needs head-on. When I am especially worn-down, I fall prey to asking questions that are not really questions. Last night, I was lying in bed wanting to go to sleep and my husband was rambling around the bedroom, putting his laundry away. I asked, "Are you going to be done soon?" What I meant was, "I want to go to bed. I would appreciate if you could do your chores tomorrow so I can turn the light out now." I asked a question that wasn't a question because it was easier than mustering the brain-power to make a clear statement of my needs. Glenn laughed and pointed out my nonquestion to me by saying he would be doing chores for several more hours. The result of asking nonquestions is generally not this humorous or positive.

To illustrate further, "Do you have to work late tonight?" isn't really a question if the asker wants their partner to be home at a certain time. When a desire is posed as a question, one of two things often happens: 1) the receiver doesn't realize it isn't a real question and provides an answer that is not satisfactory to the asker, or 2) the receiver becomes defensive. Let's pretend that Alice asked this question of her husband, Martin. If Martin thinks this is actually a genuine question, his answer might be, "Yes, I'm working late and will be home around 9:00 P.M." He would then feel blindsided when Alice bites into him with "I hate how you are never home at night!" In this case, Martin innocently answered what he thought was a true question. In the second scenario Martin might reply not to the question but to what he perceives as an accusation. Martin's defensive answer might be, "I can't help it that I have to work late! I am under a lot of pressure and you're making it worse!" Certainly, in either case, asking a nonquestion ends in negativity.

## THE MANY MEANINGS OF "DO YOU WANT TO HAVE SEX?"

Turning to a sexual example, think about a woman posing the question, "Do you feel like having sex tonight?" This nonquestion can have many possible meanings. It can even mean one thing one time and something totally different another time! This question could mean any of the following:

- *I don't want to have sex tonight because I am tired and I hope you're okay with this.*
- *I feel guilty that I have been too tired for sex lately. I want to talk about this.*
- *I hope you aren't horny, because I would love to just cuddle tonight.*
- *I am not particularly in the mood for sex, but tonight is a good opportunity since the kids are out.*
- *I don't feel interested in sex, but I know it is good when we get going. I'd like to try, but I want you to understand if it just doesn't happen tonight.*
- *I would like to have sex, but I am nervous that it won't go well since it's been so long and I'm tired.*
- *Wow! This book is working. I finally feel sexual again! Let's have sex RIGHT NOW!*

Clearly, the question "Do you want to have sex?" can mean many different things because it isn't a sincere question.

### talk *homework*

Starting today, observe how often you ask questions that aren't really questions and work to change this pattern using the skills below.

### Skill #3: Be Aware of What You Want and Your Right to Express It

Being in touch with and clearly stating one's desires are something that women don't often do. Sometimes, women are out of touch with their needs and wants. Other times, women know what they want but avoid saying it clearly. They have come to believe that directly asking for what they want, sexually or otherwise, is selfish. Yet, it is this ability to be in touch with one's needs and wants and to communicate them with clarity that is a key to mental and sexual well-being. Marlene, a thirty-nine-year-old woman with two young children, recently realized that she is much more likely to be able to relax and focus on sex if she has transition time between finishing her evening chores and engaging in sex. Once she realized this, she talked with her husband, stating her needs and wants clearly with "I" statements. She told him, "I realize that when you come up to the bedroom where I am folding laundry and ask me to have sex, it doesn't work for me. I have a hard time stopping my chores in the middle like this. I need some transition time." She and her husband were then able to engage in an effective dialogue about how to get her the transition time she needs.

Marlene became aware of the conditions or circumstances that she needed to get in the mood for sex more easily. It is also important to get in touch with what you need to make sex more enjoyable. Examples of both types of needs include:

- *I want to have sex in the morning, rather than at night when I am too tired.*
- *I want to go out to dinner and then come home and have sex.*
- *I want to find a time when the kids are not home to have sex.*
- *I want my husband to take more time with foreplay.*
- *I want my husband to give me oral sex more often.*

For now, don't evaluate how realistic what you need is. Don't think about how you could never tell your spouse these things. Just spend a few minutes brainstorming what would be ideal for you.

### talk *homework*

Stop reading and think about both what type of situations and circumstances will help you get in the mood for sex. Also, think about any explicit sexual requests that you have for your husband. Be sure to start each sentence with the word I. Jot these down and set them aside.

**meet pam,** a forty-five-year-old woman who realized that she needs her husband to use lubricant when he begins to touch her. She told her husband, "I am so tired that even when I want to have sex, I don't get wet. I find it much more enjoyable when you use lubricant when you touch me initially. It feels good and it also helps me relax and not worry about if I am going to get wet or not." Pam and her husband then had a frank discussion, resulting in agreements about who would buy the lubricants, what types of textures and smells they both preferred, and the like.

## Skill #4: Express Yourself with "I" Statements

Knowing your needs and wants is an essential first step to expressing them, but you must also learn appropriate ways of expression. Starting a sentence with the word "you" is almost guaranteed to result in an unproductive conversation. Sentences that start with the word "you" come across as accusations, and put the other person on the defensive. Contrast how you would react if your spouse said, "You never want to have sex anymore!" with "I find you really attractive and want to have sex with you and am concerned that you don't seem interested anymore." My guess is the first statement would result in you feeling attacked, defensive, or guilty. Perhaps it would signal the beginning of an argument. The latter would hopefully be the entry into a constructive dialogue.

When counseling couples, I ask them to cease using "you" statements. I ask them to use "I" statements instead. Just mastering this one skill is guaranteed to improve your general and sexual communication quite a bit! "I" statements are not selfish; quite the contrary, they are respectful of the relationship because they allow the other person to react to a real message rather than one that they have to decipher.

When opening a difficult dialogue, putting "I feel" with "I would like" is especially useful. Such a statement would go as follows: "I feel [fill in the word] when [describe situation]. I'd like [fill in blank]." An example might be, "I feel hassled when you grab my boobs when I'm doing the dishes. I would appreciate it instead if you would nuzzle my neck and even offer to do the dishes!"

Use "I" statements in as many of your conversations with as many people as possible. Learning to use "I" statements in the rest of your life will help you use them later when talking about sex. Use "I" statements with your children if you have them. Say "I want you to clean your room" instead of "You need to clean your room." Use them with your friends, substituting "Do you want to go out to lunch sometime?" with "I'd like to go to lunch with you next week if you have time." Use them for nonsexual matters with your spouse. Declare "I'd like you to try to help Scott with his math homework" rather than "Do you know anything about this new math Scott is asking me about?" There is no "you" statement in the world that can't be turned into an "I" statement.

talk *homework*

Starting today, begin as many sentences with "I" as possible. Especially start sentences with "I" that you would have previously started with "you" or phrased as a question even though it wasn't really a question. If you catch yourself asking a question that isn't a question or making a "you" statement, stop yourself and rephrase.

## Skill #5: Give Compliments and Make Loving Statements

"I love you" is an "I" statement! It is a special kind of "I" statement. It is a "soft 'I' statement." Other such statements would be "I'm having fun with you today" or "I really appreciate that you do the dinner dishes." Sexual examples of soft "I statements" would be "I love the way you touch me" or "I like how you take your time to bring me to orgasm."

Too often in long-term relationships, we stop telling each other what we like and instead spend our time focused on what we don't like or what we want to be different. We also stop saying "please" and "thank you"; sometimes, we talk to our spouses with less care and respect than we do strangers or coworkers. Stopping this downhill pattern and noticing and commenting on what you appreciate about your spouse works wonders. It helps you focus, for example, on his terrific sense of humor rather than on his annoying habit of leaving his shoes and socks in the middle of the living room. Complimenting a behavior is also likely to increase that behavior. If you take the time to appreciate the fact that he did the dishes, he is more likely to do them again. Doling out appreciation will also help your spouse feel more connected with you and is likely to result in him giving compliments in return. Focus compliments on both behaviors and on physical attributes that you like in your spouse. If you think his eyes look particularly sexy, tell him so. Remember that every day is foreplay. Appreciative and loving statements are an excellent form of foreplay.

## talk *homework*

Starting today, say at least two loving or appreciative things to your spouse each day.

## Skill #6: Use Reflections

Just as couples need to remember to say appreciative and loving things to one another, they also need to learn to have difficult dialogues. One particularly useful skill for difficult dialogues is reflection. A reflection is when you repeat back what you heard the other person say. It is best when followed by an inquiry asking if your reflection is accurate or not. It is even better when this is followed by repeated reflections and inquiries, to make certain that the listener is reacting to what is actually being said. This mode of communicating is often the first thing I teach couples that I work with.

A conversation with reflections might go as follows. Harold says, "I feel like you never want to have sex anymore." Nan would reflect, perhaps saying, "So, you think I hate sex!" Harold would clarify, saying, "No, that isn't what I am saying. I'm not assuming you hate sex. I just feel hurt that you don't seem to want to have it with me." "So, you feel upset that I don't want to have sex and think it is about you and that makes you feel hurt?" Nan would reflect. "Yes, that's right!" Harold would affirm. Nan might then say, "Well it isn't about you, it is about me." Harold would reflect, saying "So, you are saying that your lack of interest in sex isn't about me but is something in you?" "Yes," Nan would reply.

Such conversations initially feel unnatural and cumbersome, but are a very effective way to keep difficult dialogues from escalating. They enable couples to work through problems more effectively. Please remember and practice the skill of reflection the next time you have a difficult dialogue with your spouse.

## Skill #7: Find the Grain of Truth

Another key skill during a difficult discussion is to find and reflect the grain of truth in what the other person is saying. When you are in conflict with your spouse, keep in mind that there is likely some truth in what he is saying. If you can find it and acknowledge it, the disagreement will de-escalate and a solution will be arrived at more quickly. This technique reminds me of my late father-in-law. When he and my mother-in-law were fighting, he would say to himself, "This is the woman I love and respect. She is a very smart woman. There must be some truth in what she is saying. I will find it." The next time you are in the heat of battle with your husband, take a deep breath, slow down, and remember he is not the enemy and that he likely has some valid points. Nothing will defuse conflict quicker than if you or your spouse can say with sincerity, "I see your point." So, when talking about sex or any other topic, remember to look for the other person's point that has validity and let them know that you see it.

### Communication Skill #8:
### Time Your Difficult Communications Well

Timing is everything. What you have to say is not going to be heard if you say it at a lousy time. As a general rule, you should avoid having serious talks when you are at the peak of your exhaustion. In my marriage, the rule is that we don't have any serious discussions after 9 P.M., which is the time that my brain (as well as my sex drive) shuts down. Think about what time your brain shuts down. Do your best to not hold serious discussions at this time.

*I had to get comfortable talking about sex or else I wouldn't have gotten my needs met.*
—Nadine, 75

## Sex Talk

Let's talk more directly about sex talk. Perhaps this is what you were expecting this entire chapter to focus on and you are thinking, "Finally!" If so, remember that before you can talk about sex, you will need to have learned good basic communication skills. We just did this, so now let's look at five types of sex talk.

## Kitchen Table Sex Talk

Talking about sex may be difficult for you or your spouse. Many people are uncomfortable with the topic. My seventy-five-year-old friend Nadine said, "Men don't like to talk. That is why the touching is so important. I would talk during sex and say, "touch me there or here," but we hardly ever talked about sex when we weren't having it." Nadine explained that once, however, she had to talk with her husband about sex. She had to tell him that he had to slow down and take more time with foreplay. She had to tell him that women need things sexually too. Nadine says this was a hard discussion, but one that she had to have. She said, "I had to get comfortable talking about sex or else I wouldn't have gotten my needs met." Sexual problems don't solve themselves; they need to be talked about. This is true for the problem of being too tired for sex.

When working with clients, I advocate that they talk about sex as they would any other topic. It would be unthinkable to tell our spouses that talking about money or parenting made us uncomfortable and have this be accepted as a legitimate excuse to shut discussion off. Sex is a fundamental part of marriage and of life, and it is important to make it a topic for open dialogue.

When I work with couples with sexual problems, the first step is talking about the problem. Do you recall Lisa and Alex, the couple in which the man thought that women didn't like sex? Without a conversation, they could have never resolved this misunderstanding. Once they did, they continued to talk and Lisa was able to tell Alex what she likes sexually. Alex did the same. They talked and talked until talking about their sexual preferences was as comfortable as talking about their food preferences. In fact, this is the goal

I set with them. I encouraged them to learn to talk comfortably outside the bedroom and explained that this would help them to learn about each others' sexual needs and would also assist them in feeling comfortable talking during sex when needed. Lisa and Alex talked their way back into a good sex life.

Similarly, do you recall Marlene telling her spouse that she needed transition time between chores and sex? If sex was a taboo topic, she would have been unable to have this conversation. If she was unable to have this conversation, she would still be turning her husband down each time he came upstairs when she was folding laundry. Now, due to their ability to talk about sex, he comes upstairs and asks if she wants to have sex. If she does, she tells him that this sounds good but that she needs a little transition time first. Sometimes he offers to fold the laundry and she retreats to rest or read an erotic book. Sometimes she says yes and tells him she will come to get him when she is ready, after her chores are done and she has some down time. None of this could happen if they had not been able to talk about sex. Instead, they talked to successfully solve a sexual problem.

*Kitchen Table Sex Talks* are problem-solving talks that occur outside the bedroom. In fact, it is best to not bring up sexual dissatisfaction or any other difficult topic (e.g., money, children) in bed; the danger is a creating a negative association to a place that you want to be fun, exciting, and positive. It is better to have these talks in a safe, nonsexual place such as during a walk, or as the term suggests, at the kitchen table. Of course, make sure to use "I" statements and the other communication skills discussed in this chapter. Say, for example, "I think it would help me get turned on if you…" rather than "You don't seem to know how to turn me on." Likewise, remember to time your *Kitchen Table Sex Talks* well; having them five minutes before relatives arrive for a visit isn't a good time. Neither is when you are exhausted. In the final section

of this chapter, you will approach your husband to have your first
*Kitchen Table Sex Talk.*

> *Having him talk to me like this*
> *helped me realize that there was*
> *something there to be found.*
> —Kimberly, 37

### Provocative Sex Talk

While *Kitchen Table Sex Talks* are focused on dealing directly
with problems and issues, *Provocative Sex Talk* is focused on having fun. Like *Kitchen Table Sex Talks*, they also occur at nonsexual
times. *Provocative Sex Talk* is a type of everyday foreplay. Kimberly,
a thirty-seven-year-old woman, has a husband who travels a lot. He
calls her at night, after she has put the kids to bed, and sometimes
says sexually provocative things. One time he asked her where her
hands were and what her nipples looked like. Kimberly said that
while at first she just laughed, eventually she played along and "this
did something to me." For Kimberly, *Provocative Sex Talk* helps her
realize that, in her words, "there is something there to be found."

Another type of *Provocative Sex Talk* is sharing one's sexual
fantasies. Talking openly about one's fantasies is very intimate
and can bring much closeness to a couple. Also, talking about
fantasies outside of the bedroom allows couples to decide if the
sexual fantasy is something that both partners would enjoy trying.
Chapter 8 includes some resources on learning to use and share
fantasies with your spouse.

*Provocative Sex Talk* also consists of jokes and evocative hints about sex, helping to keep sexuality in the forefront of your relationship. *Provocative Sex Talk* reminds you and your husband that you are more than just two people sharing the chores and hassles of daily life. It reminds you that you have a special secret that only the two of you share. According to Dianna, "Once the subtle teasing and insinuations of sex go away, that's when you are on that slippery slope. For me, that was the nail in the coffin." Still, Dianna can take this nail out and try *Provocative Sex Talk* again. So can you.

An ideal time to experiment with *Provocative Sex Talk* is after you and your husband have had a successful sexual encounter. For example, if you have sex at night, you might want to send your husband an e-mail the next day. Perhaps something along the lines of: "I can't stop thinking of last night" or "Thinking of last night is getting me wet." Then, keep this *Provocative Sex Talk* going.

As you recover your sex drive, you may find that your first twinges of horniness occur at times when you are not yet ready to drop into bed exhausted. If this occurs, call your husband at work and tell him that you are thinking of him and would like to make love. Even though you aren't likely to be able to pull this off, putting it out there can work wonders for becoming a sexual couple again.

If you aren't yet ready for *Provocative Sex Talk*, that's okay. Just keep it in mind as something to try later. You will be reminded of this when we get to *Trysts*.

## Let's Have Sex Talk

As you will learn in the *Tryst* step, rarely do married couples, especially those with children, end up having sudden, unplanned passionate sex. This is because they have way too many other obligations and distractions. Besides, the kids are often right there! Given this, sex is often discussed first. Such discussions often begin with some kind of invitation from one partner to the other. Some couples have a secret language for such invitations. As you may recall, Lisa and Alex refer to sex as "making spaghetti." For them, an invitation might come as the coded phrase, "I'd love to have a spaghetti dinner tonight. Would you?" "Do you want to have sex?" or "Should we have sex?" are more common conversation starters. Since these are questions that aren't questions (a pitfall of communication discussed earlier), a better phrasing would be "I would like to have sex and am wondering if you are interested."

Because you generally feel too tired for sex, you likely aren't the one in your marriage initiating such invitations. Thus, it is very important that as soon as possible, you learn to accept or turn down your husband's invitations gracefully. The most graceful way to do either is with "I" statements. "I would love to have sex with you" is a loving acceptance of a husband's invitation to have sex. A graceful no might be "I love you and am attracted to you, but I am just too exhausted and distracted for it to work well. I hope we can find a time soon." Something in between might be, "I would like to give it a try, but I am pretty tired so we may end up just cuddling." The key is to use loving, "I" statements, whether saying yes or no to your husband's sexual advances. This is a type of sex talk you can begin practicing immediately.

Learning to make your own advances is also important. Don't worry if you aren't there yet. You will be by the time we get to the *Tryst* step. After reading that chapter, you may find yourself saying things along the lines of, "The kids are out, and I would like to make love while we have the house to ourselves."

### In-the-Midst Sex Talk

The media has misguided us about the importance of talk during sex. In the movies, no one talks during sex but everyone knows what to do and does it just right. In real-life sex, talking can be a powerful tool for enhancing passion and satisfaction. Talking during sex can serve many useful purposes.

#### MAKING REQUESTS

Talking during sex can include brief requests, such as the one Nadine referred to, instructing one's spouse to touch here or there, harder or lighter. "More," "Faster" "Slower" "Harder," or "Now" are words often uttered, sometimes intentionally and sometimes impulsively, during sex. This type of talk can be essential to enhancing sexual pleasure, and will be explained and practiced in more detail during the *Touch* step.

#### MAKING DECISIONS TOGETHER

Talking during sex can include making joint decisions about what you are doing, such as discussions about what position for intercourse each of you would prefer. Such discussions will go much better if you use "I" statements rather than questions that aren't questions! Instead of asking, "Do you want me to be on top?" or "What position sounds good to you?" say "I'd like you to be on top. Is this ok with you?" If you are used to having good communication and talking about sex outside of the bedroom, such discussions can go quickly during sex and any differing preferences can be easily worked out. Your husband may reply, "I prefer you be on top, but that's okay" or may counter with "I really want you to be on top" and you may say okay and climb on up. If you think this sounds unromantic, I urge you to think about how much more romantic it is than having sex that isn't enjoyable. That isn't going to do much to rev up your lacking libido!

### IMPROVING SEX AS IT IS HAPPENING

Talking about sex can also focus on what is going on and improving it. For example, a couple I worked with shared a fairly amusing, but informative, story. The woman in this couple was in the midst of a job search. During one sexual encounter, her husband noticed that she seemed distracted. He simply observed this and sought to understand it. "I notice you seem distracted and wonder what's going on," he stated. She replied in a forthright manner, telling him, "I'm really sorry. But, honestly, I can't seem to let go. I keep rewriting my résumé in my head." They then stopped for a few minutes and discussed what would help her to focus. She decided she needed a backrub since this helps her relax. Her husband gave her a massage, and she was able to let her worries go and focus on enjoying sex. Now, they use this as a quick way of conveying the notion of being distracted during sex. "Are you writing your résumé?" or "I want to have sex but I am afraid I am so stressed it will be résumé-writing sex," one of them might say. For this couple, talking during sex helped to solve a problem that was occurring in the moment, and it also gave them a special way to talk about this same type of problem in the future.

### CHECKING OUT ASSUMPTIONS

Talking during sex can also include checking out assumptions. Another couple I worked with, Jack and Anna, both had the problem of unchecked assumptions getting in their way during sex. Jack liked to receive oral sex, but worried that Anna would get tired of this. Likewise, Anna liked to receive manual stimulation but worried that Jack would get bored by doing the same thing over and over. Their unchecked assumptions created so much discomfort that by the time they came to see me, they had stopped having sex. They had tried multiple sex therapy techniques but none had worked. I advised them to check out their assumptions during sex. Anna learned to say, for example, "I am enjoying this but am afraid you are getting bored." When Jack reassured her that he wasn't, she had to learn to trust he was telling the truth. When she did, she was then able to relax and enjoy herself. As stated by Anna, "I have read every self-help book on sex there is. None of them told me I have to get my faulty assumptions out of my head and verbalize them. It has worked magic! Everyone should talk during sex."

> *It has worked magic!*
> *Everyone should talk during sex.*
> —Anna, 42

### EXPRESSING IT'S HOT AND MAKING IT HOTTER

Talking during sex can also be used to give positive feedback, or as an additional turn-on. This type of talk can be done verbally or nonverbally. Often people sigh, moan, and groan during sex. These sounds, along with heavy breathing, are a way to tell our spouses what we like. Sex sounds may also enhance our sexual pleasure, both when we make them and when we hear them. In two separate studies, both men and women reported that sex sounds were a turn-on for them. Some scientists even hypothesize that there are legitimate physiological reasons that sex sounds are a turn-on, in that they involve hyperventilation and arousal of the central nervous system. Additionally, several sex therapists and writers point out that the deeper into the sexual experience we get, the less inhibited our sex sounds may be. Recall the notion of mindful sex from the previous chapter; for some, mindful sex is noisy sex. You might want to experiment with increasing your sex sounds.

Like sex sounds, actual verbal utterances made during sex can be used to give positive feedback, or as an additional turn-on. Just telling your spouse, "That feels good," "I love the feel of your skin," "You're getting me so hot," or murmuring "mmmm" can be both reinforcing and exciting. Some women say that this kind of sex talk increases their ability to have mindful sex, since saying sexy things aloud keeps them away from having distracting thoughts; it's hard to be thinking about unpaid bills and saying sexy things at the same time. Nevertheless, women vary in what they are comfortable saying during sex. Some women like to voice their sexual fantasies during sex, to tell their partners what they are going to do to them, or to hear their partners say the same. Some women like to say or hear profane words. Other women would be uncomfortable with—or even turned off by—saying or hearing such words. Explicit talking during sex is a preference like any other; some people like it and some don't.

### After-Glow Sex Talk

Talking after sex can be a useful experience. My friend Patti has a marvelous sex life. Routinely, after sex, she and her husband discuss what has just occurred. They sometimes rate their sex, on a one-to-ten rating scale. "What was that for you?" one of them will ask. They then use this as a way to discuss what would have made it a better encounter or to revel in pride at their high scoring accomplishment. They expect to sometimes have mutually low ratings. They also expect times when one of them reports a rating of two and the other reports experiencing a nine. All this is simply material for nondefensive and open discussion.

### Sex Talk is Important Talk

My guess is that you will find some of these examples intriguing and some of them will sound a bit crazy to you. But, I hope my point is clear: sex talk is very important to a satisfying sex life and it is going to help you get your sex drive back. Talk about sex when you aren't having it. Talk about sex in the middle of having it. Talk about sex when you are done having it. The more you and your husband talk about sex, the more sexual you will feel!

## Bring Your Husband on Board

It is time to have your first *Kitchen Table Sex Talk* about your waning libido and request your husband's assistance in helping you recover it. Where you start with this dialogue will depend on a variety of factors, including how much you have already been talking about your lost libido and how solid your communication skills are in general. Of course, if you find that you are frozen with dread and can't even begin this conversation, then you need more than this book has to offer. Turn to Appendix A to find a therapist. Do the same if you try this conversation and it turns out to be an awful experience. I certainly hope this doesn't happen—and I don't think it will for the vast majority of you—but I do want to account for all possibilities.

Accounting for a variety of possibilities is why I have included several sample scripts below.

### Lead-in to Sample Scripts

First, you need to open the conversation. Try something along the lines of:

*I want to talk with you about something important to me. I hope this is a good time, but I want you to tell me if it isn't.*

*I want to talk with you about my low sex drive and a book I've been reading. I'd like to get a sitter and go out to dinner to talk about this.*

In short, make sure you are having this talk at an optimal time. And, as this talk progresses, remember to avoid making "you" statements or asking questions that aren't questions. Instead, use "I" statements.

I wish I could be with you as you have these conversations, as I am with the couples I counsel. However, I am confident you can do this! Use the scripts below as a guide to help get you started.

### Sample Script #1

*We haven't talked about this, but I know we've both noticed my lack of interest in sex lately. It has nothing to do with you or our marriage. It's because of how tired and stressed I am. I bought a book about it and think it could help. The author gives some homework assignments for us to try together. I'm hoping you're willing to do this with me. I love you and want to feel sexual again.*

### Sample Script #2

*I know we've talked before about how I'm not too interested in sex lately. I heard of a book about this and I've been reading it. It's helped me figure out what's going on. It's not about us, it's about me. It's* because I'm so tired and stressed. Apparently, women's sex drives are way more affected by stress than men's. I think this book can help me. But, I need your help too. The author recommends talking with your spouse about the problem, and she gives things for us to try together. I'd like to find a time each week to talk with you about the book and what the author suggests. Maybe I can even mark some passages in the book that I think would help for you to read. I hope you'll do this with me. I want us to have sex more often.

### Sample Script #3:

I want to talk about our sex life. I know we'd both be happier if we were having sex more often. But, I always feel so tired that I'm not interested as often as I wish I was. So, I've been reading a book about it. It's actually really common. Anyway, the author has an approach she calls the Five T's and a Bit of Spice. The T's are thinking, talking, touch, time, and trysts. I did the thinking chapter, and it's helping. Now I've read the talking chapter and I learned some communication techniques that I want us to try together.

### Sample Script #4:

I want to talk about how I'm so tired that we hardly ever have sex anymore. I don't want it to be like this. I want us to have sex more often again. So, I've been reading a book about it. It's already helped me feel better just knowing how common this is. The author has some suggestions that I think could help, but she says if they're going to work, it has to be something we do together. So I'd really like you to read the chapter I just read and then find a time to talk about it. I'd actually like to do this with the next four chapters since they have all the suggestions in them. I hope you'll do this with me. I think it would be good for us. I want to feel like I used to and have sex more often.

### Sample Script #5

*I'd like to talk with you about that book you've seen me reading. Katie said it helped her recover her drive and so I bought it to see if I could get mine back. I've learned some stuff I want to tell you about. The book talks about how we first have to learn to communicate better to get our drive back. It made me realize how we hardly ever say appreciative things to each other anymore. So, I don't know if you noticed, but I've been trying to tell you more each day how much I appreciate you. It's helped me focus on the good things about us. I'd really like if you could do this for me too. It may sound weird to you, but I'm sure it will be a good step for me in getting my sex drive back. I'd like us to try this. Actually, there are lots of things the book suggests that I would like to try, but I want to start with this one.*

Likely, none of these scripts will fit your situation exactly. Use the parts that do and also add on your own words. Remember: You don't have to address everything in this first conversation! I sincerely hope—and predict—that it will be your first of many wonderful sex talks with your husband!

### talk *homework*

Your final and very important homework for this *First-T, Talk,* is to simply open the dialogue. Have a *Kitchen Table Sex Talk* about your lost libido and your desire to regain it.

# Talk Step Wrap-Up

Good communication is the foundation of a good marriage and a good sex life. Remember the importance of asking for what you want, checking out assumptions, and working out issues as they arise. Keep in mind the notion that the purpose of disagreements is to get closer rather than to win. Practice the important communication skill of matching your verbal and nonverbal communications. Time your difficult dialogues well, and during them use reflection and work to find the grain of truth in your spouse's point-of-view. Don't ask questions that are not questions; instead get in touch with and express your needs with "I" statements. Finally, remember to say something loving and appreciate to your spouse every day. Talk about sex when you aren't having it: solve sex problems at the kitchen table. Make sexual jokes and innuendos to remind you and your husband that you are a sexual couple. Initiate and respond to sexual invitations with grace; use "I" statements for both. Talk during sex to solve problems, make decisions, check out your assumptions, give feedback, and turn up the heat. Have talking be part of the after-glow for you and your spouse. In short, talk your way back into a great sex life!

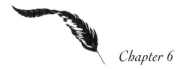

*Chapter 6*

# Energy for Life Priorities:
# Time for Tired Women

The next focus is time, something you likely feel very short of! In a survey of 2,600 women, one of the top three life concerns listed was being too busy for sex.

What do you do when you feel too busy? What do you forfeit when you are tight on time? Take a minute and think about this. Perhaps even jot down your answers.

If you are like many women, you give up what you need most. The National Sleep Foundation surveyed 1,000 women and found that 33 percent said they stop having sex with their partners when they are tight on time. Thirty-seven percent said they stop eating healthily, and 39 percent said they decrease the time that they spend with friends and family.

Such choices are detrimental to one's health and marriage and often, inconsistent with one's stated life values and goals. Many women say that their relationship with their spouse is of utmost importance to them, yet this is the first thing to go when tight on time. Even higher numbers of women seem to consider taking care of themselves as a negotiable demand.

## The Unselfish Act of Self-Care

I assume you have heard the old saying, "If Momma ain't happy, ain't nobody happy!" A related proverb is that you have to fill your pitcher before you can fill everyone else's cup. Both reflect the notion that you cannot adequately give to others if you are not taking care of yourself.

Although women often think of self-care as selfish, just the opposite is true. Being selfish is to be focused on one's own needs regardless of the needs of others. Selfish acts come at the expense of others. Self-care, on the other hand, is intentionally taking time to do something that energizes you. Self-care decreases stress and enhances physical and emotional health. Taking care of yourself will make you a better spouse, parent, worker, friend, and care-taker of aging parents.

*meet tammy,* a forty-four year old interior decorator and mother of two who recently realized how her level of self-care affected others. Her husband and children complained about how crabby and hard to live with she had become. When we examined this in therapy, Tammy admitted that her family was right—she had grown increasingly irritable at home. She also realized that this was because, in the face of stress at work, she had stopped taking her centering and energizing daily walks with her dog. Instead, she was opening the door and just letting him out, and using her usual dog-walking time to do extra work. "My not taking care of myself is bad for my husband and my kids. It's even bad for my dog!" Tammy realized. "I wish I could muster the motivation because I feel I am important enough to take care of," Tammy admitted. "But, I guess I will just be content to take care of myself for them." Tammy also noted that she now understood what people meant when they said they had stopped smoking or engaging in other unhealthy behaviors so that they could be there for others in their lives. We discussed that perhaps the motivation didn't matter—just so long as she engaged in self-care. Tammy resumed her self-care and reported that her husband, children, and dog were happier. Actually, so was she.

*My not taking care of myself is bad for my husband and my kids. It's even bad for my dog!*
—Tammy, 44

Oftentimes, busy women declare that they simply don't have time to take care of themselves. The irony is that saying there is no time to take care of yourself means that taking better care of yourself is exactly what you need to do! To recover your sex drive, you will need to start taking care of yourself.

**meet kristen,** a thirty-two-year-old client who came to me for depression. When I first introduced the concept of self-care, she said she had never heard of this before. She, like many women, had great difficulty differentiating selfish acts and acts of self-care. Still, after much cajoling, Kristen slowly gave self-care a try. She tried out a variety of activities: walking, watching movies, taking bubble baths, and participating in exercise and yoga classes. Kristen soon discovered that for her, nothing quite did the trick as much as a warm bubble bath with music and candles. I thus instructed Kristen to spend half an hour each week taking a bubble bath and experimenting with different candle scents and bubble oils. Doing this helped Kristen to focus on her own needs and to elevate them in importance. Kristen slowly added other self-care activities to her routine. She began to exercise and to take the time to eat more healthily. Soon, Kristen's depression lifted. Not surprisingly, as her depression lifted, her sex drive returned. I knew that Kristen had really embraced self-care when she told me that she gave herself a dozen roses. After accomplishing something really special in her life, she picked up the phone and ordered herself flowers!

> *My husband and I have become economic partners, co-parents, a logistical team. It leaves me dry in more ways than one.*
> —Deborah, 49

## Time Together: The Dregs of Your Day Don't Count

Do you and your spouse currently consider time with each other as something that comes after everything else? Do each of you give each other the low energy, can't-talk-to-anyone part of your day? Does your only greeting after a long day sometimes consist of a request to talk about a chore or upcoming child-related event?

Deborah is a married forty-nine-year-old woman with one teen daughter. She works two jobs to make ends meet. Earlier, Deborah was quoted as saying that her sex drive felt like a fleeting dream she was trying to recall. Deborah says that she and her husband "...are now economic partners, co-parents, a logistical team." Deborah explains that her relationship with her spouse has become "…about how are we going to make this work? How are we going to pay the bills? How are we going to orchestrate teaching our daughter to drive? Who is going to take to her to school or to her dance class?" While acknowledging that this is necessary to navigate the demands of life, Deborah says that it "leaves me dry in more ways than one." Deborah loves her husband but has no energy to interact with him at the end of the day. "I just want to destress and have time alone," Deborah explains. Deborah says that she and her husband generally watch television together, since they are both too tired to talk. The extent of their conversation is an occasional comment or two about the show they are watching. She laughingly adds, "I'm sure television isn't one of your *T*'s." Deborah sums up, with a sad look on her face, "This isn't a very sexual place to be."

## Time Means More Than Time in Bed

The story of a couple giving each other the no-energy part of their days is a common one. Another story that may feel familiar to you is Jean's. Jean doesn't feel her spouse prioritizes spending time with her, yet he still wants to have sex with her. According to Jean, "Just because you put your hand there doesn't mean it's ready. The song and dance has to start earlier in the day. The closeness doesn't start with a hand in that place. It starts with time together." Jean goes on to say that her husband is "happy when that part is happy" but that she needs more than "just my parts attended to." Jean says that time with her husband is the foreplay she needs but isn't getting. "It would have to start with some different type of time together" laments Jean. "It's not just about the bed."

### The Importance of Connected Time

Happy couples spend quality time together. They know that doing things together increases their closeness as a couple and their happiness as individuals. A close bond with your spouse decreases stress and increases feelings of well-being. The feeling that you have someone you enjoy spending time with and who is there for you even during bad times is important to your physical and emotional health. One researcher even found that being part of a loving marriage could lower blood pressure. Another study found that the less time that couples spent together, the more infrequent their sexual encounters were. Spending time together leads to feeling connected; feeling connected and having sex go hand-in-hand.

*Sex is so much better for me after we spend time together.*
—Hannah, 46

Women are especially likely to emphasize needing to feel connected to their spouses to feel sexual. Hannah is a client in her mid-forties with two teenage children and a full-time job. One night, both of her teenage boys were spending the night at friends' houses, so she and her husband decided to spend time together. They took a long walk and went out to dinner. After several hours together, Hannah felt spontaneously sexual for the first time in a long while and invited her husband to go home and make love. They did, and it was lovely. Afterwards, Hannah said to her husband, "Sex is so much better for me after we spend time together."

He asked why, and she told him it was because she felt relaxed and connected. He said that sex was better for him after spending time together also—adding with a laugh that this was because Hannah wanted to have sex. Hannah's husband was saying that he would be willing to have sex almost anytime, but that he had learned that Hannah's feeling connected was the key.

Spending time connecting with your husband is important to recovering your sex drive. But where will this time come from?

## The Paradox

"Exactly!" you may be thinking. "Where am I going to find time to spend with my husband or to take care of myself?" You are reading this book because you are too busy and tired to have sex, and now you are being told to make time for something else. That likely feels impossible, annoying, and unfair. Your irritation may increase further when you read that you need to carve this time out and plan for it. You probably feel like your life is already too tightly orchestrated. Perchance you were hoping that spontaneity would be the cure—not another demand on your time! Or, perhaps like Susan, you simply hate to plan anything in the little downtime that you have; fun, you believe, shouldn't have to be planned.

"It's a real eye roller!" is what Dianna told me when I suggested she carve out time both for herself and for her relationship. Yet, she knew it was necessary. She said it was akin to making her budget. "I can't expect my finances to be in order if I don't plan my monthly budget, and I guess I can't expect to spend time with my husband if I don't plan for it."

You have lost your sex drive because you are too busy—you aren't taking care of yourself or your relationship sufficiently. Without attending to these, you can't get your sex drive back. It's like continuing to drive your car when the low oil light is on. You will damage your engine, perhaps beyond repair. Please, don't do that to yourself or your relationship. Make the time to stop and get some oil. If you had the luxury of all the time in the world, you wouldn't need this book. You are reading this book because you want to get your sex drive back. You have to work on what has zapped it in the first place: not enough time for the things that are important to your sex drive, including yourself, your relationship and sex itself. As you read on, remember that, even though this seems paradoxical, it actually isn't. And besides, the end (feeling horny and having good sex) justifies the means (making time in an already overloaded life).

But, back to the question: where will you find this time?

## Four Steps to Finding Time

You cannot simply add in additional time to a busy day or week. There are no "extra" hours to draw from. Something else may have to go.

The first two steps to finding out what can go is examining your life priorities and comparing these to what you are spending time on. The next step is aligning your life priorities with how you spend your time. Underlying this way of proceeding is the idea that if something is a priority you need to make time for it.

If you keep finding that you don't make time for something that you say is a life priority, you will need to ask yourself why. Perhaps it isn't really important at all. Or, perhaps something else is getting in the way, such as anger or fear. My client Janice wants to get an advanced degree. She tells me that this is her most central life goal. Yet, she has said this is important to her for years and has never taken any steps toward this goal. Janice makes time for other things that are important to her. She exercises every day and meets her best friend for lunch each week. In therapy, Janice and I set several small goals to help her achieve her larger aspiration of getting an advanced degree. One week she was supposed to look at the admissions requirements for the local college and another week she agreed to talk with her husband about how they might rearrange the home responsibilities so she could go back to school. But, week after week, Janice came back without these assignments done. Finally, after becoming conscious of her repeated lack of follow-through, Janice had the insight that two things were getting in her way. First, she was afraid of failure. Second, she realized that as long as she didn't have her degree, she could stay angry at her husband for his earlier failure to support her education. As long as she remained without her degree, she held some power over her husband through holding on to her anger. Janice had to let go of both her anger and her fear before she could pursue her life priority. She then had to dedicate time for school, shoving other responsibilities aside. A life priority can't be something you give lip-service to; it has to be something for which you make time.

## Step #1: Set Your Priorities

This activity involves setting your current life goals. I purposefully use the word "current" because life goals continually change. Psychologists often recommend evaluating your life goals on a yearly basis.

Take out a piece of paper. Record today's date. Then, write "My Life Priorities" at the top. Because of your focus on regaining your sex drive, write "Have a good sex life" on your list. Then, write the following other two items: "Have a good marriage" and "Take care of myself." Bluntly, if you are not willing to put these items on your list of life priorities, you might as well put this book down. Reading this book isn't going to help you reignite your sex drive unless you truly begin to think of self-care, your relationship, and sex as top life priorities. You are reading this book because getting your sex drive back is important to you. To recover your libido, you will need to put your marriage, sex, and yourself on your priority list—and you will then need to spend time on these priorities.

Before turning to spending time on these priorities, take a moment to add two other items to your list. These can be something you are already doing and want to keep doing, or they can entail something you would like to do that you are not currently doing. These goals can revolve around people or groups of people. An example of a goal in this category would be "Be a good mother." Goals can be work-related, such as "Become a partner in my law firm" or "Open my own clothing alteration business." Goals can be about your health and well-being, such as "Exercise daily" or "Lose fifteen pounds." All of these can be current top life priorities. When you are done, you will have a list of five life priorities, of which your sex life, your marriage, and taking care of yourself are the top three.

After you have written your list, look at each of the items. My guess is that some are more easily measurable than others. Perhaps having a good sex life seems a bit vague to you. What behaviors can you use to measure this? For this goal, you might include both indicators of quality such as the percentage of time you have an orgasm and your ideal frequency. In terms of your ideal frequency, there is no right answer here. Think about what would be ideal for you. We will come back to this answer later. For now, however, if frequency of sex is part of how you will measure what it means to have a good sex life, then write down the number of times per week you would ideally like to have sex. Likewise, write down anything else that helps you define what it means to have a good sex life. Additionally, do this for any of your five goals that are vague. For each one, list two to five concrete behaviors by which you can measure this goal. If one of your goals is "Be a good mother," you might write: do not raise my voice; spend time each day focused on my children; set firm limits with my children, or the like.

At this point, you should have a list of your current top five life goals, as well as ways to measure the accomplishment of these goals. Now, let's continue with matching your goals with the way you spend your time.

### Step #2: Assess Your Current Time

Think about how you spend your time in two categories: inflexible and flexible. Other words that capture this are non-negotiable and negotiable. Inflexible activities can be those you choose to do or those dictated by others; they can be set in stone because you make it so or because someone else makes it so. Probably the best example of the latter is a job with set hours. Another example is a monthly parent association meeting for your child's sport team. Self-imposed inflexible time includes those things that you make time for that you are rigid about. My client, Cynthia, sets her alarm for 5:30 A.M. each day and meditates for fifteen minutes. Nothing but an absolute emergency or serious illness gets in her way. My friend, Jennifer, jogs every day without fail, although she varies the time of day depending on other activities. Still, this is inflexible time in that she always fits it in.

Flexible time, on the other hand, includes those activities that you choose to do. It also includes activities that you must engage in that can vary in how much time you spend on them. Examples of chosen activities include surfing the web for enjoyment and watching television. Examples of the other type of flexible time—

those things you must do but can adjust the time you spend doing them—include cooking, grooming, and even laundry. You have to eat, but you can spend twenty minutes to two or more hours on food preparation. You have to wash your hair, but you can spend an hour styling it or you get a lower maintenance hair cut that takes less time to style. You have to wash your underwear, but you can vary the time you spend putting it away. Like my mother, you can fold it neatly and put it in a drawer or like my sister you can toss it unfolded into the dresser. Or, you can do what I do: leave it unfolded in the laundry basket and let the family pick their panties from there each day. In short, we all have to eat, wash our hair, and clean our underwear—but the time we spend getting there can vary. There is some flexibility built into these "must-do" activities.

Activities in both the flexible and inflexible categories can be enjoyable, neutral, or aversive. Just because something is set in stone doesn't mean you don't enjoy it. Likewise, just because you choose to spend time on something doesn't mean you enjoy it or that it is time well spent.

Take a moment to examine your time in accordance with these categories. You can either just think about this or you can write it down. Consider the ways you spend your time that are inflexible because they are either self- or other-imposed. Then, think of all the ways that you spend your time that have some flexibility to them, either because you can vary the time you spend on them or because you are engaging in these activities by choice.

### Step #3: Creative Time Shifting

Then, think about the five life priorities you just set and the notion that if something is a life priority, you must dedicate time to it. To truly prioritize something, you have to begin to think of the time that you spend on it as inflexible, even if it is self-imposed inflexibility. Successful exercisers don't schedule anything during their exercise hours. Successful writers don't give up their writing hours. People who get enough sleep don't stay up late, even when they have something left undone. If something is a priority, you must not consider it as something that you can let go of when other things interfere. Life priorities must translate into time that you spend that is non-negotiable.

Still, the problem of finding such time in an already busy life remains. One obvious place is to take the time spent on an activity that you are choosing to spend time on that doesn't coincide with your life priorities.

### *meet kathleen,* a mother of two school-age children

with a part-time job as a real estate agent. Her work hours are set around her children's school schedule; while her children are in school, she works. She also uses this time to see friends, perhaps meeting them for lunch or coffee. When I met Kathleen, she was feeling emotionally and sexually depleted. Our first task was to put self-care on her priority list, and have her spend time on this. As we examined how she was spending her time, she realized that her encounters with certain friends left her feeling more stressed and depleted than when she had begun. Slowly, she cut back on her time with these obligation-friends, and used the time on self-care. She started meditating and exercising instead of eating lunch with her energy-zapping friends.

To make time for herself, Kathleen cut out something that she was doing by choice. Another option is to use less time doing those activities that you have to do, but for which the time spent is not set in stone. To illustrate, my client Jasmine used to spend thirty minutes a day putting on makeup. She now spends ten minutes and uses the other twenty for exercise. To do this, Jasmine had to decide that exercise was more important than makeup and then to spend time on what was important to her.

### *meet rachel,* who came to therapy for exhaustion and anxiety. Her anxiety was so consuming that she wasn't sleeping and wasn't having sex with her husband. One of the sources of Rachel's anxiety was caring for her ill, aging parents. When her parents became ill and Rachel assumed their care, the thing that she gave up was her own self-care. Through therapy, Rachel realized that she had given up what was essential. She realized that unless she was willing to care for herself, she could not expect her anxiety to dissipate. After a thorough examination of how she could rearrange her time, Rachel decided to stop cooking and delivering meals for her parents. Instead, she paid for meals-on-wheels and spent the time she had used cooking for herself. Her anxiety soon dissipated. Her sex drive eventually returned.

Another client, Mellissa, realized she was spending about thirty minutes each night tired and engaged in household puttering chores that weren't really necessary. Her husband was doing the same thing. So, now, at 10:00 each night, she and her husband both call it quits and get in bed together. Some nights they read and go to sleep. Other nights, they cuddle. Other nights, they have sex. Either way, these are thirty minutes that are much better spent than they previously were.

The point of the stories you just read is that even in the busiest of lives, a tiny bit of time can be carved out for the life priorities of taking care of yourself and spending time with your spouse. Take some time to think about creative ways that you could shift your time around to make time for your life priorities. Write it down if it helps you commit to truly spending your time differently.

### Step #4: *Live the Commitment*

Spending time on what is important (you, your relationship, and sex) doesn't just happen. It takes the action of prioritizing what is important, closely examining how you are currently spending time, and then finding ways to re-arrange your time to make room for priorities. The final step entails making this commitment to yourself and sticking to it. The last step is to put your time where your priorities are. The rest of this chapter will help you do this. The rest of this chapter is about living the commitment of spending time on yourself and your relationship.

## Committing to Self-Care

Just what activities women consider self-nurturing varies. Some women find time with friends nurturing and others find time alone nurturing. Some women find walking nurturing while others find sitting quietly nurturing. My mother enjoys getting manicures. My sister, on the other hand, finds sitting for a half hour while someone does her nails stressful. She would rather spend this time exercising.

Just as what each woman will find nurturing will vary, so will just how much self-care a woman needs vary. A psychologist colleague of mine encourages her clients to figure out the minimum time they need for self-care on a daily, weekly, monthly, and yearly basis. I tend to help my clients think in terms of days and weeks. I encourage clients to engage in at least some self-care on a daily or weekly basis. I encourage them to find an activity that is enjoyable and revitalizing.

Randi is a full-time working mom of two children under the age of eighteen months. She barely has enough time to go to the bathroom, let alone engage in self-care. She has found something nurturing, however, that takes less than two minutes a day. A friend gave her several inspirational books, most of them divided into quotes or very short stories. She reads one story each morning. Randi knows that as her children grow, she will have time for other self-care activities but for now, she does these one-minute reads and they help her to remember that her own needs and thoughts are still important.

Self-care activities don't need to take a lot of time and they don't need to be elaborate. They should, however, be healthy. Using excess amounts of alcohol, drugs, or food as self-care is actually self-destructive in the long run. Certainly, this doesn't mean that a self-care routine can't ever involve food or alcohol. However, if a client requires these to relax, I would be concerned.

When deciding what would be a good way to care for yourself, one thing to consider is whether there are activities you used to enjoy that you have given up. My client April used to love painting but had slowly stopped doing so because she spends most of her time working and raising three children. For April, then, carving out time to paint each week made for a splendid form of self-care. Another client, Nellie, loved to sing; she had sung in choirs as a teen but hadn't sung in years. She bought herself a karaoke machine and spent time singing. Other ways that clients and friends have found to take care of themselves include the following:

- *Taking a walk*
- *Gardening*
- *Reading*
- *Taking a class at the local college*
- *Taking a yoga class*
- *Meditation*

- *Watching a favorite TV show with no interruptions*
- *Going to a movie alone*
- *Spending time with a friend*
- *Getting a manicure or pedicure*
- *Dancing*
- *Masturbating*
- *Getting a massage*

The latter three self-care activities are particularly good for recovering one's sex drive. Dancing can be very erotic; some women take belly- or pole-dancing classes as a way to both take care of themselves and to rev up their sex drive. Masturbation also counts as a way to both take care of your own needs and to charge your motor for sex with your spouse. Likewise, the skin-on-skin contact in massage can help to increase feelings of well being and sexual desire. Certainly, you can go for a professional massage, but this is also something you and your husband can do for one another. Trading five minute back rubs or foot rubs daily is a way to get self-care needs met, while also enhancing closeness and intimacy with your partner.

Despite these double benefits of masturbation and massage, as far as your sex drive goes, there is one self-care strategy that is the best of all.

**meet jackie,** a thirty-five-year-old single, full-time working mother of two boys under age ten. Finding time to exercise is a challenge. But, because Jackie knows that if she doesn't exercise she becomes anxious and impatient, she has come to prioritize exercise. She gets up a half hour before her children each morning and runs on her treadmill. Committing to a daily exercise program takes a great deal of effort, but it is worth it. Jackie stays fairly centered, despite the demands of her life. And, it's no coincidence that Jackie never complains of a waning libido. She is a highly sexual woman, whether she has a current lover or not.

## Work Out to Rev Up

Exercise is the #1 self-care strategy for both your physical and emotional health—and importantly, it is among the best ways to rev up your sex drive as well!

Exercise can help to fix some of the things that may be zapping your drive in the first place. Exercise is a very effective stress reducer. Studies show that a daily cardiovascular exercise routine reduces symptoms of anxiety, and being less anxious will help you feel more sexual. Exercise, especially when done in the morning or afternoon, will also help you sleep better at night, and being better rested will give you more energy for sex. In addition, when you commit to an exercise program, you are engaging in a clear action to improve your life. This can enhance your positive feelings about yourself and the belief that you have the power to improve your life—feelings that are likely to feed your waning libido. Exercise will also help you feel better about your body, and thus help increase your motivation for, and comfort with, sex.

Exercise also helps you get in touch with your body and its sensations, and the more in touch you are with your body the more likely you are to feel sexual. You can also bolster this effect by focusing on sexual thoughts and feelings as you exercise. Do you recall my friend Teresa, who notices sexuality and sensuality in all that she does? She consciously does this during her daily exercise. When walking, she purposefully notices her nipples rubbing on her shirt and focuses on the positive feeling.

When swimming, she attends to the feeling of the water swirling around her vagina. You may want to give this a try the next time you exercise.

Even if you don't focus on sexual feelings as you exercise, working out is still likely to enhance your sex life. A study found that women aged forty-five to fifty-five who exercise report higher levels of sexual satisfaction than women who don't exercise. In another study, women who exercised were more sexually aroused after watching an erotic film than women who didn't exercise. It may be because exercise increases the blood flow all over the body or it may be because exercise increases energy in general. Regardless of the underlying reason, your sex drive is likely to be turned up by exercise.

For exercise to be beneficial, it must become a regular habit. It also must be something that you can feasibly fit into your life and that you enjoy. Perhaps this is an early morning walk. Perhaps it is an exercise tape or class. Maybe it is a jog on the street or on a treadmill. How about swimming or an aerobics or jazzercise class?

Some people prefer to exercise alone and some people prefer to have a workout partner. In one study, couples that worked out together were more likely to stick to it than were individuals who worked out without their spouses. Some couples also report that sexual energy can arise when working out with each other. On the other hand, some women find exercising to be their alone-time haven, as well as great problem-solving time. Teresa tells me that it is during her daily solo-exercise that she often discovers solutions to things she has been wrestling with, both in her professional and personal life. She says this further enhances her view of exercise as time well-spent. Whether done alone or together, exercise is medicine for your stress and your sex drive.

*meet* *heather,* a client whose story demonstrates the power of exercise. Heather is a forty-two-year-old stay-at-home, divorced mother of two sons. Heather has pervasive self-doubt and very low energy. She finds it a constant challenge to stay on top of all the things that she needs to do to maintain her house and care for her children. Heather also says that there was a time in her life she exercised and she knows she "should do this" again. She says she knows that exercise helps to combat her depression, but that she still doesn't do it. Heather and I talked about the concept of dividing time into flexible and inflexible categories, and I initially encouraged her to think of exercise time—even five minutes a day—as non-negotiable time. Heather said that while she understood inflexible time could be something she was choosing, this way of thinking didn't work for her. She said thinking of anything as inflexible made her feel trapped. She said that for her the focus had to be on the choice part of the equation. "If I think of exercise as something I want to do, as something in my choice time category, then that will help," Heather told me. We found a five-minute block of time for starters and Heather would tell herself, "I am going to choose to exercise now." The results were almost miraculous. Just five minutes of exercise a day for a week lifted Heather's spirits. The next week she increased to seven minutes, the next to ten and so on, until she was consistently exercising half hour almost every day. Not surprisingly, Heather's energy increased and her depression decreased.

Except in cases where it is prohibited for medical reasons, I encourage every client who comes to me for depression, anxiety, and/or a decreased libido to engage in daily exercise. In almost every case, it contributes to recovery. Now it's time for you to do the same.

### time *homework*

If you do not already engage in regular exercise, think about what exercise would work for your lifestyle. Look at your schedule and find a way to commit to exercise. The eventual goal is to exercise a minimum of twenty minutes a day, three days a week. More is even better. But it is fine to start with a modest commitment, as Heather did, and build up to this goal. START TODAY!

## You Can Do It! Take the Final Step!

Perhaps you are taken aback at this homework, in that you are being asked to make a serious commitment and a permanent lifestyle change. Please know that I wouldn't ask you to do this if it wasn't of critical importance to regaining your sex drive. You are too tired for sex because you are not prioritizing yourself or your health. You are too tired for sex because you are stressed by multiple pressures. Taking care of yourself through exercise is going to decrease your stress and increase your sex drive. While you learned in Chapter 3 that sex improves your health, the reverse is also true: taking care of your health, through exercise, improves your sex life. It may take you several months to be convinced of this, but if you stick with it, you will be.

### Time Homework Talk Tip

To find a way to fit exercise in your life, you may need to talk with your spouse. You may need assistance carving out time for this. Or, perhaps this is something that you want to suggest doing together. Either way, unless you can add in exercise at a time that doesn't involve coordination with your spouse, such as a lunch hour at work, you will need to discuss this. Use "I" statements to tell your spouse that you want to begin a regular exercise program and need his support. Make concrete suggestions and requests for ways that he can help you fit exercise into your life or for the two of you to exercise together. An example conversation starter is: *I want to start exercising and I need your help finding a specific time each day I can do this.*

### An Overall Healthy Lifestyle

Along with your exercise regimen, I also encourage you to get enough sleep and eat healthily. Lack of sleep is directly related to lack of libido. Likewise, good nutritional habits will enhance your health and thus your sex drive. In addition, you are strongly urged to engage in other self-care activities as often as possible. Look at the list of self-care activities again. Which appeal to you? Try to find time for some of these as well, or simply keep them on your radar and look for opportunities to engage in them.

### An Unwavering Commitment

As you go through the days in your busy and demanding life, remember that self-care is now one of your top life priorities! Remember also that it is critical to make time for what we say is important to us. You have now made a commitment to self-care. Please make it an unwavering one. Stay steadfast to making time for one of your top priorities: You.

# Committing to Relationship Time

Now that you have committed to self-care, you are ready to do the same thing for something else of critical importance on your priority list: your relationship. There are multiple ways to spend time connecting with your spouse. In the next chapter, we will focus on spending time touching your spouse. For now, our focus is on nonsexual, nonphysical connecting. But, any touching or hugging or kissing that you do during these times is definitely going to enhance your connection and put you a step ahead on your path to passion. Likewise, when spending time with your spouse, remember to say affectionate and appreciative things to him. Engaging in *Provocative Sex Talk* can also be an added bonus during time together. Say something sexual, for example, while taking a hike.

Below is a list of of ideas for ways to spend quality time with your spouse. Some are quick and some are more time-intensive.

- *Share the highlights of your day together.*
- *Take a walk together.*
- *Read a book out loud together.*
- *Take a shower or bath together.*
- *Go out on an evening date together.*
- *Go on a weekend get-a-way together.*
- *Rent a movie and watch it together.*
- *Go on a drive in the country together.*
- *Put on music and slow dance together.*
- *Take a ballroom dance class together.*
- *Listen to music together.*
- *Play a board game or a card game together.*
- *Go on a bike ride together.*

- *Garden together.*
- *Go on a picnic together.*
- *Exercise together.*
- *Work on an enjoyable home improvement project together.*

The critical word is *together*. Find something that you and your spouse both enjoy and spend time doing it together. Ideally, you will spend some time each day together (e.g., five minutes talking about your days) and some more intensive time (e.g., a date) each week. But, even if this goal is too lofty for now, the key is to begin to make spending connected time with your spouse a priority.

To illustrate, let's return to Alex and Lisa. Although they have been married more than twenty-five years, Alex and Lisa share few interests in common. Partly because of this, over the years their lives have became one of parallel existence rather than of connectedness. However, they both wanted to feel more connected to one another, emotionally and sexually. When we first tried exercises to help them sexually connect, these exercises met with failure. Eventually, we realized that this was because they first needed to start simply by spending nonsexual connected time together.

Lisa and Alex agreed on a weekly date, for which they would take turns planning the activities. Because of their diverse interests and both of their tendencies to avoid talking about their own needs, the two rules for dates were: 1) it had to be fun for the planner, and 2) it couldn't be an activity that the other would dislike. They agreed that dates would occur every Saturday night. They also separated their dates from sex. They found that if they didn't, their dates included unspoken tension about whether they were going to have sex or not and this detracted from their enjoyment of spending quality time together.

Lisa and Alex were creative about their Saturday nights together. One date planned by Lisa was a home-cooked gourmet dinner followed by poetry reading. Dates planned by Alex included hikes in the woods and teaching Lisa to prepare the deer he had recently hunted for meat. As Lisa and Alex engaged in these dates, they found that they had more in common than they thought. Lisa enjoyed preparing the deer and Alex enjoyed the poetry. They also began to slowly spend more spontaneous time together, although this was not part of their prescribed homework. Most importantly, their connectedness increased and this was in large part responsible for their eventual return to sexuality together.

Another factor that may have helped contribute to Lisa and Alex's revitalized sex life was the novelty of the activities they engaged in together. Research shows that sexual attraction peaks among couples after doing new and challenging activities together. While white-water rafting and mountain climbing would certainly count, so would novel activities that are easier to achieve. Sarah and Jim found that going dancing instead of out to dinner helped to rev up their libidos. Emily and Todd found that going to a comedy club instead of a movie brought them enhanced energy. Think about novel ways you could spend time with your spouse.

### talk *homework*

Talk with your spouse about the importance of spending nonsexual, connected time together. Share with him that such time is important for you in recovering your sex drive. Tell him that you would like to commit to spending such time together. Remember to use "I" statements. Say for example, *"I want to spend more time with you. Spending more time together would help me feel more sexual again."* Discuss with your spouse ways to spend time together. Talk about what you used to do together that you both enjoyed and express your current ideas for time together while remaining open to his ideas. Say for example, *"I would like for us to spend time together. I want to talk about some fun new things we can try together."* Or, *"I would like to spend more time with you. I'd love to spend five minutes each night completely focused on hearing something important from each other's days. I'd also like to hire a sitter and start going out one night each week."* Your goal is to open this conversation and then to begin to consistently spend nonsexual, connected time with your spouse in a way that works for the two of you.

## One More Time-Related Relationship Tip: Organizing Time

Constant chatter about who does what leaves little time for any other conversation. In addition, the typical dynamic is the wife ends up being the CEO of the household; she tracks what needs to be done and when. She may then become resentful that she has to do all this organizing work, her anger escalating if she asks her husband to do something and he doesn't do it. The husband, on the other hand, often feels like his wife is constantly nagging him and telling him what to do.

Some method of clearly dividing up the chores is strongly recommended. Such division is needed for the standard weekly or monthly chores, as well as the daily hassles that arise. This will help avoid miscommunication and resentment about who does what. Such resentments are definitely sex drive zappers!

Do you recall Deborah, who was quoted earlier saying that her relationship with her spouse had become all about how to navigate their shared responsibilities? Deborah also lamented the daily phone call on the way home from work to discuss what to do about dinner. She told me, "If we spent half as much time talking about what we should do about sex as what we should do about dinner, we would be in good shape!" Deborah and her husband could actually free up some time for other activities if they planned their dinners, or other joint stressors, in advance.

> *If we spent half as much time talking about what we should do about sex as what we should do about dinner, we would be in good shape!*
> —Deborah, 49

Kelly and Wayne did just this. Kelly stays home with her two children and Wayne is an attorney. When I first met them in therapy, they had many built-up resentments. One of Kelly's biggest complaints was that Wayne assumed she was always available to take care of the children, even during Wayne's nonworking hours. She felt disrespected by this assumption. Wayne, on the other hand, reported that he didn't know that Kelly needed things to be different. While therapy revealed that Wayne needed an attitude adjustment about the importance of his needs versus Kelly's and that Kelly needed better communication skills, another fix was simpler. Specifically, Kelly and Wayne needed to synch their busy schedules to avoid misunderstandings and resentments over time issues. Kelly and Wayne went with a high-tech option of synchronized computer schedules and Blackberries.

Lisa and Alex went with a lower-tech option. They now have a weekly meeting with paper and pencil to coordinate schedules. These weekly meetings help them to stay committed to the notion that time together is a top priority. Their planning includes who is doing what (such as grocery shopping and cooking dinner), each of their self-care times, their nonsexual date, and their weekly tryst. Lisa and Alex coordinate their schedules to do exactly what this chapter advocates that you do: make yourself and your relationship priorities and spend time on them.

## Time Step Wrap-Up

Self-care is not a self-centered act: It benefits both you and your relationships. It's also great for your sex drive! Spending time on your marriage is also important to your health and well-being, as well as a necessity to recover your sex drive. But, just any time won't do—it has to be quality connected time. On the surface, it might seem like a paradox that someone as busy and tired as you would be asked to find more time in your schedule to recover your sex drive. But, deeper examination shows that this isn't really a contradiction at all. To recover your sex drive, you have to put three very important things on your list of life priorities: yourself, your relationship, and sex. You then need to spend time on these priorities. Hopefully, you have now been able to carve out such time by examining how you currently spend your time and creatively moving things around a bit. Most important, you have committed to a lifestyle change that includes both exercise and quality time with your spouse. Live this commitment! In short, spend time on what is most essential to you—and your sex drive will follow.

*Chapter 7*

# From Ice Cold to Steamy Hot:
# Touch for Tired Women

We are born with the need for skin-to-skin contact. Studies conducted in orphanages and hospitals reveal that infants who aren't touched lose weight, become ill, and even die. On the other hand, premature babies who are provided with touch gain weight faster, cry less, and have improved pulse and respiration rates.

Your sex drive mirrors these findings. Without touch, your sex drive shrivels and dies. Conversely, loving, sexual, and affectionate touch can all help to rejuvenate your libido. Rarely will a tired woman initiate sex or respond with ready passion to a spouse's advances if there has not been connected touching throughout the day and week. As stated by Nadine, my seventy-five-year-old friend who has had a satisfying sex life over the course of her fifty-five-year marriage, "You need to be defrosted. If you haven't been touched all day and go to bed at night, you're an ice cube. It's hard to go from an ice cube to boiling water. Being touched during the day warms you up." But, just any touch won't do. Some touch warms you up and some touch frosts you further!

## Not While I'm Doing the Dishes!

Have you ever been in the kitchen, perhaps doing the dishes, and your husband comes up and gropes your rear end? If you are like most busy, tired women, your reaction won't be instant pleasure. You will be annoyed. Why? Isn't this the same person whose touch, or even gaze, used to send shivers up your spine and tingles down to your vagina? Isn't this the same person whose kitchen-groping used to result in playfulness? Dianna described her change in reaction as a "sad little journey." She explained that when her husband used to come up from behind and grab her breasts, she would turn around and engage with him and play back. Later, she said, this turned into a smiling rebuff. "Come on honey, I'm trying to do the dishes," she would say. Sometime later, her reaction was a scowl and total rejection. Now, she realizes with some sadness, "He doesn't even try anymore," and "I've become one of those women I never wanted to be."

*You need to be defrosted. If you haven't been touched all day and go to bed at night, you're an ice cube. It's hard to go from an ice cube to boiling water. Being touched during the day warms you up.*
—Nadine, 75

Why does this story sound familiar to so many women? Why does your husband copping a feel while you are cooking or doing the dishes result in irritation? According to Susan, a client who came to therapy with her husband Jack, it is because "He only pays attention to me when he wants sex." According to Amy, another client, "It feels too abrupt and devoid of affection. It turns me off and not on."

But, what do husbands say? A session with Fred and Paula is particularly enlightening. Paula was lamenting that she wished Fred wouldn't grope her while she did the dinner dishes. She explained that this was a turn-off and that a much more effective turn-on would be a gentle kiss on her neck and an offer to help with the chores. To illustrate her point, Paula asked Fred, "How would you feel if you were fixing the car and I came up and grabbed your penis?" "I would love it!" he replied.

Fred's quick and honest answer led to a useful discussion about why Fred groped Paula and the type of touch they both craved from one another. Fred wanted more sex, but just as importantly, he also missed the sexual playfulness of their earlier years. He was using this indirect, joking method of touch to keep him from feeling vulnerable. This way, if Paula rebuffed him, he could tell himself it didn't matter since he was just messing around. Fred's touch had evolved from loving and sexually provocative to teasing fumbling. Fred learned that this was not an effective way to get closer with Paula or to get her interested in sex. Paula, in turn, realized that Fred's groping was actually an indirect invitation to be close and to touch, maybe even to have sex sometime later. Paula learned that Fred did indeed understand that, unlike in their pre-child years, she couldn't just stop doing the dishes to make out and maybe have sex. He wasn't expecting sex on the spot; he just wanted to be a close and sexual couple. In her exhausted annoyance, Paula had lost sight of this. In the end, Fred agreed not to grope Paula but instead to be more sexually provocative and also to initiate sex through more affectionate and sensual touch. Paula, in turn, agreed that when Fred approached her in the kitchen the next time, instead of reacting with quick, rejecting anger she would take a deep breath and respond with playfulness or affectionate touch. You might want to try the same and see what happens. You also might want to have a talk with your husband like Fred and Paula had about the kitchen sink groping. But, first, you need to take a much simpler step toward getting the touch you need.

## Watch and Discover

Your first step to getting the kind of touch you need is to take one day (or better yet, one weekday and one weekend day) to monitor what type of touch you are giving and getting. Don't do anything to change what you or your spouse is doing. Instead, simply observe it. How often do you touch your spouse in an affectionate way? How often do you touch him in a sexually provocative way? How about in a teasing way? How often does your spouse touch you in these same ways and how do these types of touch make you feel?

As you observed yourself and your spouse, you may have discovered how infrequently the both of you show love and affection through touch. On the other hand, you may have noticed that you touch affectionately but not sexually. Like Dianna you may have discovered that "hugs are all that is left." If this is the case, you are already a step ahead in the program. Still, it will benefit you to further increase your level of touch or to experiment with new ways of touching one another affectionately. It will benefit you because affectionate touch is the building block for tired women to rekindle their desire.

# The Wordless Language of Love

Affectionate touch is basic to a loving, sexual, relationship. Touching your spouse with affection is a powerful way to say, "I love you." Recall from the communication chapter that when our verbal and nonverbal behaviors conflict, we give most weight to the nonverbal ones. The same applies to the language of love. Saying "I love you" without words can be even more compelling than saying it with words. Conveying love and affection through touch can be the most potent, even intoxicating, message of all.

No wonder studies show that one of the predictors of a woman's marital satisfaction is how affectionate her husband is. Affection also bolsters physical health. Perhaps you recall that hugging decreases blood pressure. In one study, women sat very close to their spouses, talked with them for ten minutes, and then hugged them. Even this short-lived affection lowered blood pressure. Affectionate touch is a healthy—and health-enhancing—way of communicating love.

## *A Language for All Ages*

Did you ever notice how young couples in love touch each other almost constantly? Often people say things like, "Isn't that sweet?" or, "They are so adorable." Likewise, have you ever seen an elderly couple holding hands or showing other forms of physical affection? Have you smiled at the sight? Have you hoped that you and your spouse would be like that in your later years? The reality is that you can't expect to be affectionate later if you aren't now. Affection is an important cornerstone of all phases of marriage. It's time to start talking this language now.

## The Many Words of This Silent Language

There are countless ways to show affection or love through touch. Here are some of the many ways:

- *Holding hands*
- *Massaging necks, shoulders, and backs*
- *Giving each other full-body nonsexual massages*
- *Rubbing each others' feet*
- *Hugging each other*
- *Sitting close enough that you are in physical contact*
- *Holding one another*
- *Playing footsie with each other*
- *Walking arm in arm*
- *Resting your hand on your spouse's leg or arm*
- *Cuddling with one another*
- *Rubbing your face against your spouse's face*
- *Sniffing each other on the face, neck, or shoulders*

The possibilities are endless. Can you think of other ways of showing affection to your spouse? How about ways you would like him to show affection to you?

## The Way They Like It and Like You Mean It

When working with individuals who have marriage concerns, I often instruct them to touch their spouses affectionately more often. Frequently, this touch is reciprocated without any discussion: as one spouse ups the affection, so does the other in response. Likewise, when working with a couple, I give them an important first assignment: each should initiate affectionate touch five times a day. Before embarking on this homework, I have the couple discuss what type of affectionate touch they like the best. Some people prefer a shoulder rub whereas others prefer a hug. It's good to know what type of affectionate touch you favor, as well as to know what your spouse likes. Often in relationships, we tend to give what *we* want—rather than finding out what the other person wants and giving them that.

Likewise, sometimes we get stuck in our patterns of giving affectionate touch; we touch in ways that seem perfunctory and devoid of real affection. Sam and Ellie often held hands but it didn't really feel loving or connected. It felt habitual and emotionless. What helped them was to hold hands differently—to use their thumbs to caress one another as they held hands or to hold their hands in new and different positions. Even this small change prompted them to notice and appreciate each other's touch more.

### Start "Talking" Now

It is important that you start speaking the silent language of love now. To regain your sex drive, you and your husband will need to increase the amount of meaningful affectionate touch in your marriage. You can do this without discussing it, and see if your spouse follows in kind. If not, you can address it with him more directly. Or, you can address it with him directly from the start.

### touch *homework (choice a)*

Start touching your spouse affectionately several times each day. If you already engage in affectionate touch, increase the amount of this kind of touch and vary it in terms of type of touch to make sure that it is meaningful and connected, affectionate touch.

## touch *homework (choice b )*

Talk with your spouse about the importance of affectionate touch to reviving your sex drive. Tell him that you would like for both of you to touch each other in an affectionate way several times a day, or that you would like to vary and enhance the intensity and connectedness of the type of affection you already share. Say for example, *"I would like us to touch each other affectionately more every day"* or, *"I would like us to purposefully touch each other with genuine affection every day"* as an opener for this discussion. Discuss the types of affectionate touch you both like. Then, be sure to remember to touch your husband in the way he likes.

### More Silent Love Language: Talking with Your Gaze

Up until now we have been focused on physical touch. But, talking with your eyes is another powerful way to speak love without words. The notion of speaking love with one's eyes is often used at couple's relationship retreats, where "soul gazing" is practiced. During soul gazing, partners look deeply into one another's eyes. As they do, they have some form of physical contact such as holding hands or putting their hands over one another's hearts. As couples look deeply into one another's eyes, they are instructed to focus on communicating love through their eyes. Sometimes they are instructed to coordinate breathing. If this activity appeals to you, explain it to your husband and tell him you would like to give it a try.

If soul gazing doesn't appeal to you, you may still want to extract the basic principle: a loving gaze. Remember to actually look into your partner's eyes. In the early stages of a relationship, couples report spending time gazing into one another's eyes. Later, we are often so busy running around that we don't stop to look anymore. Try to slow down enough to consciously, and lovingly, look into your husband's eyes, if for only a few seconds. Make a real connection, even if fleeting, with your eyes.

In accordance with the notion that much of this book is best digested and tried in chunks, I encourage you to put this book down and work on communicating love and affection, using both your hands and your eyes, for a week before moving on.

# No-End-Goal Touching

Hopefully, you are now enjoying giving and receiving love and affection through touch and gaze. Continuing this affectionate touch is paramount to recovering your sex drive. Now, it is time to crank up the heat a notch. It is time to add in *No-End-Goal Touching*.

## How it Works: The Pleasure of No Pressure

To understand the premise of *No-End-Goal-Touching*, take a moment and think back to when you were a virgin, before you first engaged in intercourse. Do you remember what my mother's generation would call "heavy petting" or what my children's generation call "making out"? Can you bring to mind a sexual encounter from these days? When I recently asked Dianna to recall such a time, her wistful reply was "It was wonderful." Like Dianna, perhaps you recall becoming wet and excited, even though you knew the evening would not end in intercourse. After all, reminisced Dianna, "What could we really do in a car parked in my parent's driveway?" She wondered, "Perhaps some of the excitement was the lack of pressure itself." Like Dianna, do you remember a make-out session that resulted in moist underwear and a throbbing vagina? Perhaps you even came home and masturbated. If you had no one to confide in, you may have even wondered if your degree of lubrication and excitement was normal. Did all girls get this hot?

> *What could we really do in a car parked in my parent's driveway? Perhaps some of the excitement was the lack of pressure itself.*
> —Dianna, 54

*No-End-Goal Touching* is designed to warm you up. It is designed, quite literally, to get your vaginal juices flowing again. Its ability to get you excited lies in the fact that there is no pressure to actually have sex. Non-pressured sexuality is probably the exact opposite of the pattern that you and your husband currently find yourselves stuck in.

Likely, you have responded to your husband's invitations for sex by saying, "No, I am too tired" a number of times. If your spouse is like the husbands of many tired women, he has become discouraged by this. He has slowly ceased to touch you affectionately. He has stopped reaching out to you as often, or even at all, with sexually provocative touch. This decreased affection and eroticism has likely further dampened your sexual desire. It has also contributed to turning sexuality into something that is cut off from the rest of your life. If you are like most tired women and their husbands, sex has become an all-or-nothing proposition. You probably currently hesitate to start anything that you can't finish. This is quite problematic because it leaves you crawling into bed at night exhausted and, as seventy-five-year-old Nadine said earlier, "cold as ice" as well. There has been no "defrosting." *No-End-Goal-Touching* can fix this.

## The Napkin Dropping Trick

For *No-End-Goal Touching* to be effective, you have to engage in it at times or in places where sex is out of the question. This works both because of the lack of pressure and because our sexual desire often increases when there are barriers to fully satisfying it.

You can suggestively caress your husband's inner thigh under the table during a dinner with friends. He can do the same for you, perhaps even allowing his hands to covertly rub your vaginal lips through your pants. My friend Evelyn's husband "accidentally" drops his napkin when out to dinner with friends; when he reaches or crawls under the table to get it he finds a way to slip Evelyn a very sexually erotic touch, particularly if she is wearing a skirt. One time Evelyn anticipated that Bill would do this and the surprise was his when he found that she wasn't wearing underwear under her long, flowing skirt. This same couple has been known to pretend they are cold at the movie theater, putting a coat across their laps and engaging in extraordinarily provocative touching of one another—touching that doesn't lead to intercourse in the movie theater but gets both of their juices flowing for a later time.

Certainly, all non-demand touching doesn't need to be quite this intensely sexual. You can have a five minute make-out session on the couch while your child is taking a bath. You can nuzzle one another's ears. You can shower together in the morning and engage in some sensual and lathery touch that doesn't lead to intercourse. You can slip your hand in your husband's pants pocket and give his thigh a squeeze. He can stroke your rear-end or breasts, for just a few seconds. No matter what you do, the point is to integrate suggestive touching into your daily life.

## What Turns Up Your Heat?

Before engaging in *No-End-Goal Touching*, you need to know what type of sexual touch you and your partner find most arousing. Just as the type of affectionate touch that individuals prefer varies, so does the type of sexually provocative, non-demand touch. Do you get excited when your partner nuzzles your ear or neck? Caresses your thigh? Kisses you passionately? As was the case with affectionate touch, it's important to know what type of sexually provocative touch you and your husband each prefer. Knowing this will prevent you both from making the all-too common mistake of giving what we ourselves desire—rather than what our partners crave.

When in the midst of *No-End-Goal Touching*, remember to use the mindfulness focus you learned in the *Thoughts* step. Fully immerse in the pleasure for these few minutes. Also, communicate what you like, either during or after the encounter. After a particularly provocative make-out session, you can let your husband know that it worked and that your vagina is throbbing. Or, you can simply tell him how nice that felt.

## What About Finishing the Deed?

Despite its effectiveness to help build passion, *No-End-Goal-Touching* is often met with skepticism. The concern centers on the tension between sexually provocative touch and "finishing the deed," or having intercourse. The husbands of women who have lost their sex drive sometimes fear becoming further sexually frustrated by these exercises.

In therapy, my job is to convince these husbands that *No-End-Goal Touching* could be frustrating in the short run, but is likely to get their sexual needs met better in the long run. I tell them that, believe it or not, they will most likely come to enjoy *No-End-Goal Touching*. I remind them that even in the most sexually active part of their relationship, not all touch led immediately to intercourse or orgasm. I remind them that in the past, a hot session of lovemaking would often be followed by provocative touch and talk the next day, including at times when sex was impossible. The old pattern was that a hot romp in the sack would lead to *Provocative Sex Talk* and *No-End-Goal Touching*, both of which would keep the arousal high until another hot session of lovemaking. I explain that we have to start this cycle back up again and that a good place to start is with *No-End-Goal Touching*. I can't converse with your husband, but you can have him read these paragraphs or using your newfound communication skills, you can explain this to him yourself.

### touch *homework*

Talk with your spouse about the importance of integrating sexual touch into your lives. Tell him that you would like to give this a try. Tell him that you would like to add this type of touch to your daily life together. Say for example, *"The book I am reading recommends that we get sexual at times that we can't actually have sex. I would love to do this."* As you discuss this exercise, be open to discussing any concerns he has about increased sexual frustration and share with him the notion that even if this exercise is frustrating in the short term, it will likely result in more sex in the future. As you explain *No-End-Goal Touching* to him, open a dialogue about what kinds of sexually provocative touch you both like the most. Then, continue to give your affectionate touches, but also add in this type of touch, ideally on a daily basis.

........................................................................................................................

While you are starting with once-a-day *No-End-Goal Touching*, this type of touch builds upon itself. It is so much fun that you are likely to naturally increase the frequency as you learn to savor these hot moments.

## Playtime

Another exercise sex therapists sometimes recommend is taking turns pleasuring one another. This homework revolves around a series of turn-taking exercises often recommended for couples that have significant anxiety around intercourse. For couples dealing with this and other potentially serious relationship and sexual concerns, this tends to be a cumbersome exercise that is best done as a homework assignment while in therapy. However, its basic principle is quite useful for women who feel too tired for sex and is thus explained here. The idea is to take turns playing with one another's bodies. It is best if playtime includes a focus on whole-body stimulation and is taken slowly. The idea is to give each other pleasure, without intercourse. During playtime, one partner pleasures the other, with the partner being pleased under no obligation to reciprocate or to reach orgasm. It is this lack of pressure for intercourse and orgasm, as well as the non-mutuality, that makes this exercise so effective. The giver can learn what it feels like to give pleasure and the receiver can fully relax and revel in her own pleasure without worrying about if it is time to do something for her partner or if she is expected to orgasm soon.

This playtime can come in several varieties. For example, your husband could pleasure you and receive nothing from you in return. You could do the same for him at another time. Or, you could both take turns pleasing each other, in the same evening.

Playtime will help you get over the idea that every sexual encounter has to be equally pleasurable for both partners. This is a false belief that can get in the way of the give-and-take that is part of any good relationship, including a sexual one.

## Self-Pleasure

Another important way to get your sexual juices flowing is through masturbation. Some women used to masturbate frequently, but now feel even too exhausted for this. Sandra describes masturbation as "another relic of my sexual past."

*Masturbation is another relic of my sexual past.*
—Sandra, 51

You can't just wait until you feel horny to masturbate. If you do, you may never masturbate. While horniness used to be the signal that it was time to masturbate, you need to reverse this equation. You need to masturbate to get horny. Instead of waiting to pleasure yourself when you feel sexual desire, you can create sexual desire by touching yourself. You can also masturbate to refresh your memory of all the benefits of sex. In a survey of more than 2,000 women from their teens through their nineties, many reported masturbating to relax, to get to sleep, or to relieve menstrual cramps.

Masturbation is also a good time to practice mindful sex. Practicing a total immersion in the physical sensations during masturbation can help you achieve this state more quickly during sex with your partner. Masturbation is also good time to rediscover the old ways you used to like to receive pleasure or to experiment with new ways to excite yourself. You can touch yourself in new ways, with different degrees of pressure, in new places or in new positions. You can try reading erotica or watching an arousing movie before masturbation. You can buy different lubricants and discover what you like and don't like. You can try making different sex sounds and see if any get you aroused. Some women like to experiment with a variety of vibrators. The goal is to pleasure yourself and to pay attention to what works best for you. You can use what you learn simply to enjoy yourself, but also importantly as knowledge to enhance your relationship with your spouse. You could tell him about your new methods, or show him. If you don't feel comfortable with this, don't worry. Just turning up your own sex drive a notch through masturbation will help.

### touch *homework*

Find some time (even just five minutes a week) to touch yourself in a sexual way. You don't need to have orgasm as a goal. Simply experiment with ways of touching yourself that bring arousal and pleasure.

What you may find is that you get aroused in ways that are new or different. Or, you may discover that some of your old standards do the trick. Another important discovery might be that touch can lead to sexual desire, rather than needing to feel desire before engaging in touch. Or, maybe you already knew this, but need to think of it in a different way. The next section will help you with this.

# Getting in the Mood: Not the Same as Duty Sex

If you are like many tired women, you have been having sex when you are "not in the mood" but once it gets going it works well. Afterwards, you may think or say things along the lines of "That was good. We should do that more often." But, still, you lament not being in the mood and this lesson is quickly forgotten, until the next time you force yourself to have sex without first having the physical ache of desire. You think of this in a downbeat way. You think of this as forcing yourself to have sex. You talk of having duty sex. Duty sex starts and ends without physical desire. But, not all sex that starts with no desire ends this same way. Some sex starts dry and ends in intense sexual excitement, even orgasm. This is because of the reversed equation.

## *The Reversed Equation*

In your younger years, your sequence of sexual activity was:

Physical Desire → Sexual Activity → Sexual Excitement/ Orgasm.

This is what I call the "Feel Horny, Have Sex" order of events. This is what you are hoping to reclaim. You want to have physical desire lead to sexual touch. While the techniques in this book are aimed at this goal, it is important for you to understand that there is also another solution you can employ. This method involves using your psychological desire for sex (a desire that has hopefully been enhanced by doing your homework!) to propel you to engage in sexual activity and to allow this sexual activity to get you horny.

This alternate sequence of events is as follows:

Psychological Desire for Sex → Sexual Activity → Physical Desire → Continued Sexual Activity → Sexual Excitement /Orgasm.

This is what I will call the "Have Sex, Feel Horny" or the "Touch to Desire" order of events. This is where you have sexual encounters to get horny rather than waiting to be horny to have a sexual encounter. In metaphorical terms, this is akin to knowing that your car can be cold when you start it, but that it will warm up while you drive. You can still experience a very pleasant drive, even in winter. When explaining this to my client Rose, she also used a transportation metaphor. "Oh, I understand. Sometimes a leap of faith is the only available form of transportation." Rose went on to say that "Feeling confident that sex will be good once it gets going could propel me to have it, even when I'm not in the mood."

*Feeling confident that sex will be good once it gets going could propel me to have it, even when I'm not in the mood.*
—Rose, 44

## Be Proud of Yourself

If Rose has sex when she isn't in the mood—and if it is good sex—I hope she will feel pleased with herself! And I hope you do the same. Rather than continuing to think of the good sex you have as duty sex, another option is to view it in a positive light. Feel pleased with yourself for having sex to get horny, rather than lamenting what is wrong with you.

If you do this, you won't be alone. Two studies found that many women who lose their sex drive do not feel bothered by this. A very recent study led by a Massachusetts General Hospital physician surveyed about 32,000 women whose ages ranged from eighteen to older than 100. Findings indicated that 43 percent of the women had some kind of sexual problem, including 39 percent who said they had issues with low sexual desire. But, only 12 percent of the women were distressed about their sexual problem. While this study didn't examine how these women had come to feel unbothered, perhaps it was because they didn't allow their lack of sex drive to interfere with having a marvelous sex life.

While this sounds like a contradiction, it's not. In fact, many of you are already are doing this. You are already using your psychological motivation to have sex. You are using touch to get you excited. Keep doing this and add in a new mantra. Tell yourself, "I am happy with myself for making sex a priority," "I'm proud of myself for being so motivated to have sex," or something along these lines that works for you.

Thinking this way will help you recover your drive, because it is another form of positive thinking and because it will propel you to have sex, an act which itself revs up your libido. This new way of thinking will also help you to maintain a great sex life through the inevitable ups and downs of your sex drive.

### If It Is Fun, It's Not Duty Sex

The main point is that great sex doesn't always have to start with physical desire. Just because it doesn't start with physical desire doesn't mean it is duty sex. This is the difference between "It was awesome and I'm going to make sure to do that again soon!" and "I am glad I got that over with for the week." Using the "Crockpot Formula" will make it much more likely that you'll react positively.

## The "Crockpot Formula"

Not enjoying sex due to a husband's lack of good sexual technique is different than being too tired for sex. Still, your husband's sexual techniques and your ability to give him feedback about them deserve additional attention. How much time your husband takes with foreplay and his specific way of touching during foreplay are especially important.

### Your Hot Button: Let's Call It Sex

The traditional definition of foreplay is the caressing that takes place before intercourse. Such wording implies that touching is useful only as a lead-in to the main event, with the main event being intercourse. Given that most men orgasm during intercourse and that, according to the Hite Report, 70 percent of women *don't* orgasm during intercourse, this is a male-defined way of talking about sex. Some sex experts, and some women I talk with, say it works best if the woman can have an orgasm separate from intercourse. A few go further to say that this works best if the woman's orgasm occurs before intercourse. If these women were defining the words, the clitoral caressing (and orgasm) that occurs before intercourse would be called sex and intercourse would be called post-play. Sex expert Lori Buckley prefers the term "sex play" to foreplay, pointing out that clitoral stimulation (by oneself, one's partner, or a vibrator) can occur before, during, after—or even instead of—intercourse.

This is not to say that women don't like intercourse. Lots of women enjoy intercourse tremendously. It is just that the vast majority of women require clitoral stimulation to orgasm. For women, the orgasm "hot button" is the clitoris. The clitoris has more nerve endings than anywhere else in the body. Learning this helped one of my very religious clients get comfortable with asking her husband to stimulate her clitoris. "After all," she said, "I think my clitoris must be God's gift for me. He put all those nerve endings there for a reason."

*I think my clitoris must be God's gift for me.*
*He put all those nerve endings there for a reason.*
—Natalie, 38

During intercourse, the clitoris is only indirectly stimulated and this is why only a minority of women orgasm through penetration alone. Those women who do orgasm through penetration alone often say they do so in the woman-on-top position; this may be because of the friction of rubbing the clitoris against one's partner's abdomen or the shaft of his penis. Another theory is that women who have orgasms during intercourse have clitorises that are closer to their vagina than those who do not. The bottom line is that in order for a woman to reach orgasm, she generally must have her clitoris in contact with something and it must be stimulated.

Despite the paramount role of the clitoris in women's orgasms, sex experts are quick to tell you not to ignore other parts of your anatomy. Many women report that they receive great pleasure from having their breasts caressed. Others report feeling positive erotic sensations in the upper front wall of the vagina, the location known as the "G Spot." Still, many sex therapists and the majority of women will tell you that for the most reliable and intense sexual pleasure, women need men to take time stimulating their clitoris.

> *I told him that he needed to take a lot more time with me and slow down. I told him no more "wham bam thank you ma'am." After that, we had a wonderful sex life for the rest of our marriage.*
> —Nadine, 75

How much time? There is great variability among women. Likewise, an individual woman herself will vary, depending on many things. Among these are her level of exhaustion and her ability to focus and have mindful sex. Still, averages are interesting. On average, men take four minutes to reach orgasm, once they begin intercourse. Women take somewhere around eleven minutes and this is not eleven minutes of intercourse. It is eleven minutes of stimulation. Not all women know this. Even fewer men seem to know this. What's more, women often don't tell men this. Women don't always tell their husbands that they need time to get aroused or how to arouse them.

## Tell Him You Are a Slow Cooker

Jean has been married twenty-six years and she has never told her spouse directly what she needs. She says that lately he has been more focused on this, because of his awareness of her attraction to another man and his fear of losing her. He now tells her that he wants her "to be as finished as I am." But, Jean says, "He is ready to begin to be intimate at ten or eleven at night and I don't even want to get into talking about mechanics at that point. I just want to get it over with and get to sleep." Jean emphasizes this point further, "Sure, I could tell him to do this or do that. But, by the time he is home and ready, I don't want to bother." Jean also says that she was raised in a very prudish household and isn't all that comfortable talking directly about sex. "I don't even know how I would explain it to him."

The best way I've heard this explained was by Lana, a woman in her fifties who, despite a full-time job as a school teacher and a part-time job as a manicurist, has a very satisfying sex life. She said, "This is because Brian knows that men are microwaves and women are crockpots, and he tells me to take all the time in the world to get warmed up." This echoes the sentiment of Nadine, my seventy-five-year-old friend quoted earlier about being warmed up through affectionate touch. Nadine educated her husband early in their marriage about what she needed. "I told him that he needed to take a lot more time with me and slow down. I told him no more wham bam thank you ma'am. After that, we had a wonderful sex life for the rest of our marriage," says Nadine. Both Nadine's husband and Lana's husband learned that women take longer to become sexually aroused than do men.

If you're tired and stressed-out, it's important that your husband understands it will likely take more time for you to get aroused. It takes time to let go of stress and focus on physical feelings and sensations. If your husband doesn't know that you are a slow cooker, I encourage you to find a way to tell him this.

### Tell Him What Ingredients Work Best

You will also benefit greatly from telling your husband about the way you like to be touched or what turns you on. Knowing what you like and being able to communicate this is perhaps *the most important tip* for sexual satisfaction. All of the information about women's arousal presented above was based on averages. That means that not all women fit these patterns. Knowing what you like and telling your husband this is of critical importance. Telling him once isn't sufficient either, because the type of clitoral stimulation that women need to orgasm can change from one sexual encounter to another. For some women or during some sexual encounters, too much direct clitoral stimulation can become uncomfortable. To receive the type of stimulation you want, you can say "move your hand here or there" or provide specific instructions or requests ("softer please"). You can also communicate your desires by guiding your husband's hands the way you want them to go.

Although it doesn't eliminate the need for talking during sex, it is also very useful have an explicit sexual discussion about what you like and want over coffee or dinner. For this *Kitchen Table Sex Talk*, it might help to take out the list you developed in the *Talk* step about both the conditions you need to make sex more optimal and explicit sexual requests that you have. While talking about sex is something that many people find awkward or difficult, it is critical. That is why *Talk* was the foundational *T*. It's time to make your bed rock with the bedrock of communication.

*He knows that men are microwaves and women are crockpots, and he tells me to take all the time in the world to get warmed up.*
—Lana, 57

touch *homework*

Talk about Touch. Talk with your husband about any of the following that you think would enhance your sex life: being a crockpot, ways to warm you up, the type of sexual touch you find most arousing, the conditions you need to make sex most optimal, or any other specific sexual requests that you have.

Please have this talk now, but anticipate having more discussions after you check out all the spicy ways to heat up your sex life that are the focus of the next chapter!

***meet wanda,*** a thirty-eight-year-old nurse who recently told her husband about the crockpot metaphor. She also told him that most women needed an average of eleven minutes of clitoral stimulation. Then, the next time they made love, she reminded him with a grin, "Remember, I need my full eleven minutes!" Her husband responded with seriousness, telling her to "Take as much time as you need." This helped Wanda to relax and her relaxation resulted in her enjoying sex more than usual and having a wonderful orgasm. In fact, Wanda actually came quicker than she normally did because she wasn't feeling pressured about or focused on how long it was taking.

## Touch Step Wrap-Up

You NEED affectionate and sexual touch on a daily basis to recover your sex drive and to keep it alive. Affectionate and sexual touch shouldn't be limited to the bedroom. Such touch needs to be fully integrated into your life and your relationship. That way, it becomes a natural and enjoyable part of your inter-action with your spouse. You and your husband need to learn to touch each other affectionately several times a day. Slowing down enough to look into each other's eyes is also important. In other words, you and your husband need to take time to speak the powerful and silent language of love on a daily basis. You need to let go of the myth that all sexual touch must end in intercourse. Instead, you need to engage in provocative touch, especially at times and in situations when there is no way you could actually "finish the deed." To get your sexual juices flowing, make this *No-End-Goal Touching* a part of your daily routine. Try revving your sex drive up further with playtime; doing so will help you shatter the myth that every sexual encounter needs to be equally as pleasurable for both people. Also, please remember that just because you start a sexual encounter with no interest doesn't mean that it is duty sex. You can start a sexual encounter with little or no physical desire, and end up having great sex. You can use touch to get you in the mood. Do this and pat yourself on the back! To make sure that sex is great—whether it starts with physical desire or not—tell your husband that you are a slow cooker. Explain to him how women, especially tired women, need a lot of foreplay. Tell him about your hot button, your clitoris, and how you like to be touched. Keep telling him. Talk with your husband all about the touch you need and then revel in the feeling of his hands caressing your body. In short, allow affectionate and sexual touch to keep things steamy!

*Chapter 8*

# Spice It Up with Novelty

Some people lose their interest in sex due to boredom or to the repetitiveness of doing the same old thing sexually time after time. In fact, sometimes people are bored and aren't even aware of it. Some experts claim when they hear couples say that they don't have time for sex, they take it as a sign of boredom. The reasoning is that we find time for things that interest us, but we don't for things that don't interest us. There is a thin line between being too tired for sex and being tired of the *same-old* sex. Exhaustion and boredom can have the same effect: They both make you want to go to sleep!

Therefore, doing novel things sexually may increase your libido. This relates to the principle of habituation. Habituation is when you decrease or stop responding to something due to repeated exposure. For example, if you hang a new picture in your house, for a while you will find yourself continually looking at it and noticing it. But, as time goes by, you won't give it any special notice. You will have habituated to it. Sometimes medications stop working due to habituation to them. Habituation may be the reason menopausal women in new relationships are more likely to report having a high sex drive, whereas those in longer-term relationships are more likely to report a decreased sex drive. It also helps explain why our sex drives seem to be the highest in the early stages of a relationship: We haven't yet habituated. Trying new things is likely to decrease your habituation and thus, increase your sex drive.

Think of the ideas in this chapter as different spices on a spice rack. The spices are the things you might want to experiment with to liven up your sex life. The rack is the way to think about these spices.

## The Spice Rack:
## The Way to Approach Ideas

The spice rack is the structure or framework holding the different spicy ideas together. It includes the notion that there is no right or wrong to sexual preferences as long as no one is being coerced or doing something they find aversive. As you examine the suggestions, remember to use your own inner compass. If an idea sounds intriguing to you, try it. If it sounds repulsive, don't do it. If you are a bit nervous about engaging in something new and stretching your sexual boundaries, you are urged to push through the apprehension and give it a go. You can certainly stop whatever you are trying out at any point. Importantly, remember to communicate your preferences, reactions, and ideas to your husband. As an example, if you want to try having intercourse in a new position, find a way to tell your husband this. If he says yes, but in the midst of this position, you find yourself in pain or turned off, tell him so and stop doing whatever makes you uncomfortable.

Julie credits her satisfying sex life during more than twenty-five years of marriage to being willing to try new things and to talk about them. Julie says, "The things we try don't always work out, but we have the attitude that we will try and see. We always talk about it beforehand. Some of it works and some of it doesn't. And, even if it doesn't, we can still get closer and enjoy a good laugh together." Like Julie, as you read the spicy ideas in this chapter, approach it with the framework of being open to new ideas, listening to your reactions and feelings, and keeping good communication skills as a cornerstone.

> *The things we try don't always work out, but we have the attitude that we will try and see. We always talk about it beforehand.*
> —Julie, 58

## Spices: Ideas to Jazz Up Your Sex Life

Continuing with the image of spices on a rack, the spices are some things you may want to try to heat up your sex life. Taking this one step further, the *Five T's* of the treatment program (of which you have already completed *Four T's*) are the food that you need to sustain yourself and the ideas here are the flavors you can sprinkle on to enhance the food. Some people prefer to hold the jalapeño peppers and others ask for extra. The spices range from simple to exotic. You can try all of them. Or, you can try just one simple one to see how adding novelty increases your energy for sex.

## Play with Toys

Women have shown an increased interest in sex toys in recent years. Perhaps the most well-known sex toy is the vibrator. Women vary in terms of their interest in vibrators. Some have never used a vibrator and have no interest in doing so, some have one all-purpose vibrator, and others have a variety of types and styles of vibrators. Some women use their vibrators alone and others ask their husbands to stimulate them with a vibrator. Some do both.

Often women and their partners worry that a vibrator will take the place of sex they have together. As stated by Jean, "I wonder if too much of that battery-operated thing might cause the opposite effect of improving passion with a human. But then again, it may improve the tired part." There is no evidence that the use of vibrators decreases women's interest in sex with partners. As is the case with masturbation without a vibrator, just the opposite may occur. Many therapists and many women will tell you that their vibrating buddies increase their sex drive. This makes sense, given that sexual stimulation makes one want more stimulation.

There are many different makes and models of vibrators to choose from. Most vibrators are focused on stimulating the "hot button," the clitoris. Some are hand-held and some are strap-on. Some of the strap-on varieties even have a remote control button, so you (or your partner) can discretely stimulate yourself anytime and anyplace. Some vibrators are designed to reach the clitoris more easily during intercourse. There are also vibrators designed to reach the G Spot. Vibrators come in a wide range of styles.

### WHERE'S THE TOY STORE?

If you are interested in trying out a vibrator, or seeing what other types of sex toys are available, a good place to start your exploration is a reputable store. To learn more about what to look for in a sex shop and for a listing of good or unique shops, you might also want to check out Corey Silverberg's "Sex Shop Hall of Fame." Go to *About.com* and plug this article title into the search field. Two excellent shops with online shopping options are Good Vibrations (*www.goodvibes.com*) and My Pleasure (*www.mypleasure.com*). Both sites offer a variety of vibrators and other sex toys. Both also have excellent sex education sections. Another terrific site offering both sex education and sex toys is the store that is associated with the Sinclair Institute, a company focused on enhancing relationships through sex. Go to the Sinclair Institute website (*www.Sinclair Institute.com*) and click on *"The Store"* to check it out.

Another option worthy of mention is Passion Parties. These are parties for women that feature sex toys. It's the erotic version of a Tupperware party. Anita, a fifty-four-year-old acquaintance of mine, is a Passion Party hostess. She reports that these parties are both educational and lots of fun; the women who attend them end up sharing some intimate stories and details of their lives, as well as a lot of laughs. Such parties also focus the thoughts of those who attend them on sex—something you already know is helpful from the *Thoughts* step. You can find out more by going to *www.passionparties.com*. This site also has an online store for women who want to buy sex toys without going to a party.

### HOW DOES THIS TOY WORK?

The *My Pleasure* website has a great deal of enormously helpful information on picking out sex toys. The Sinclair Institute store has a video titled, *Toys for Better Sex*. This educational video is geared to teach couples how to introduce sex toys into their relationships to increase intimacy and mutual pleasure. In this video, loving couples demonstrate uses of sex toys. Also available at the Sinclair Institute store, Volume 3 of *The Better Sex Video Series: Sexplorations* includes discussions and demonstrations on sex toys.

### spice *homework*

If you have never tried a vibrator or other sex toy, consider whether this is something that appeals to you. If you have tried a vibrator or other sex toy and liked it, think about trying a different one. To decide, you could take a look at one of the websites mentioned above.

### Go to Sex Class

Watching an instructional video on sex can be a great way to spice up your sex life. Such videos teach new activities and skills and can also be arousing to watch. An excellent resource is Sex Smart Films (*www.sexsmartfilms.com*). This site is run by a certified sex educator and a member of the National Advisory Council on Sexual Health. Some free films are available at this site, but most are offered to download for a fee. They offer films on a variety of topics including, for example, masturbation and the G Spot. A highlight is a seven-part series that guides couples through turn-taking exercises that emphasize learning to pleasure one another and to communicate with each other while pleasuring. These exercises correspond to the notion of Playtime from the *Touch* step. Another great resource for educational sex videos is the Sinclair Institute, which offers almost 100 instructional videos covering a wide array of topics. Perhaps their most well-known video is the one mentioned above; this three-volume video covers several topics, including human sexual anatomy, the G Spot, erotic massage; oral sex, erotic talk, erotic dance; sexual fantasies, masturbation, anal sex, role-playing, and sensual touch. A small sampling of some other videos available include: *Couples Guide to Great Sex Over 40, The Art of Oral Sex, Introduction to Erotic Massage, Unlocking the Secrets of the G Spot,* and *The Erotic Guide to Sexual Fantasies for Lovers.* While a few of the videos are designed specifically without explicit nudity or sexual scenes (e.g., *Sex After Fifty, The Art of Seduction (Non-Explicit),* and *Five Steps to Sensational SEX (Non-Explicit),* most contain erotic scenes of real couples demonstrating techniques, as well as information provided by sex experts. As such, as is also true of the material available for download at SexSmart Films, most videos are both instructional and erotic and arousing to watch.

Such instructional videos are fun to watch together. Solo watching is also an option. Trudy is a twenty-nine-year-old woman who is married to her high school boyfriend, whom she met at age fifteen. She says that they both know very little about sex and in fact, just learned about the clitoris recently. Trudy was thrilled to learn about these instructional videos, although she says she would be too embarrassed to watch them with her husband. She and her husband plan to watch them separately and then discuss them together. Either watched alone or together, these videos are an excellent way to learn new things about sex and to spice up one's sex life. Written sex manuals can also help you and your husband learn new things about sex; the ones I recommend most highly are listed in the Additional Resources section.

## Play a Sexy Game

Another way to inject some spice into your sex life is to play a sexy board game. A great variety of games can be found at both the Sinclair Institute store and at My Pleasure. As an example of the more than twenty games available at the Sinclair Institute store, in the couple's *Fantasy and Romance Game*, players roll the die, move spaces, and then perform the romantic or sexual activity indicated on the board. At My Pleasure there is a game called *Discover Your Lover* that guides couples to try some new ways of touching one another, as well as to talk about sexual topics in a deep and meaningful way. Another game, *Truth or Dare* mimics the game that you may have played as a teen. The truth cards guide couples to talk about sexual matters while the dare cards lead couples to try out different sexual activities with one another. Games can be an effective way to give you and your husband ideas and permission to explore new things without the embarrassment that can sometimes come from suggesting something new oneself.

## Moisturize

Many tired women have difficulty with lubrication, either due to menopause, exhaustion, or both. Lubricants can be useful when the Touch → Desire order of events is in play. If one is engaging in touching as a prelude to feeling desire, then lubricants will jumpstart that desire. Being touched with lubricants is going to be more pleasurable than being touched when dry. The feeling of lubrication itself can be stimulating.

One way to add some novelty to your sex life is to experiment with different lubricants. There are silicone lubricants and water-based lubricants. Silicone lubricants are generally slippery and long lasting. Water-based lubricants give a feeling more similar to a woman's natural lubrication. Women who are prone to yeast infections will want to look for glycerin-free lubricants. Lubricants can also be found in a variety of flavors. Some lubricants heat or cool to the touch. A few are designed to increase sexual pleasure. While lubricants can be found in almost any drug store or grocery store, a wider variety can be found in sex stores.

*meet amanda,* a fifty-one year old woman who says she is too tired for sex, although she almost always enjoys it once she and her husband get going. Still, she wanted to reclaim her sex drive and so worked through the steps in this *Five T's Plus a Bit of Spice* treatment program. She was especially intrigued when she found out about lubricants. She said that she and her husband had been "using the same old goopy one for years." She didn't know others even existed. She was surprised to learn that she could find a variety in her local grocery store. The next time she went grocery shopping, she bought five different varieties. She reported, "Just buying them made me more motivated to have sex because I wanted to see what they felt like." She also found one she really liked. "I LOVE the *K-Y Yours and Mine!*" She says she can't imagine ever getting tired of this, but has seen the power of trying something new. "So, while this is going to be my new staple, I will still try new brands once in a while." She laughingly adds, "I also found a *K-Y* variety pack, and I gave it to all my friends for Christmas."

### spice *homework*

The next time you are at the grocery store, drug store, or general department store, stop by the aisle where they sell lubricants. If trying one appeals to you, go ahead and buy it.

### Stretch Your Sexual Agility

Trying intercourse in new positions can also add new excitement to your sex life. If this interests you, your own creativity can be your guide. The position and manner in which you masturbate can also be a way to scout out a new position. Try finding a sex position that allows you to take advantage of this. For example, if you masturbate on your stomach but usually have sex on your back, try out a position in which you can be on your stomach while you or your husband stimulates you.

Alternatively, there's no shortage of books, websites, card decks, and videos to help you discover new positions. One particularly tasteful book is Alex Comfort's *Sexual Positions (Joy of Sex)* book. One educational yet explicit (i.e., it contains pictures of real people) website is *www.goodtoknow.co.uk/relationships*. This website has a large section on sexual positions, with pictures and descriptions of each.

Good Vibrations has a store section dedicated to bedroom furniture, designed to inspire new positions. The Sinclair Institute store has an entire store section dedicated to new positions. They offer several excellent videos on sexual positions as well as sex restraints, sex swings, and furniture specifically designed for sex called *Liberators*. This dense foam furniture is available in a variety of shapes and is suitable for couples that want to try something unique, as well as for couples with physical limitations. Certainly, the types of positions that are feasible change as couples age. Our sexual agility is not going to be the same at sixty-five, with a back or knee problem, as it was at twenty, without any such problems. Volume 4 of the Sinclair Institute's *Better Sex Video Series Six-Volume Collection* deals with how sex furniture can help couples overcome such physical limitations.

## KAMA SUTRA POSITIONS

The Kama Sutra is an ancient Indian text made up of several sections, including one that describes and illustrates several different sexual positions. Although centuries old, many couples still find the sexual positions quite interesting today. My Pleasure, Good Vibrations, and the Sinclair Institute store all offer a variety of Kama Sutra products. Just go to these websites and enter Kama Sutra into the search field, and you will find a variety of books, DVDs, and games to choose from. Also, the website, *www.good toknow.co.uk/relationships*, includes pictures of real couples demonstrating a variety of Kama Sutra positions.

## *Make It a Spiritual Experience*

Tantric sex has gained popularity as something new to try, especially for couples in long-term, committed relationships. Although Tantra is an ancient religious philosophy, it has been adapted into modern, Western thought as a form of sacred sex. In its Western version, Tantric sex is said to bring couples to a more intimate and spiritual connection. Some of the basic principles of Tantric sex were part of the treatment program you have been working on with this book, including a focus on non-goal oriented sex, taking foreplay slowly and luxuriously, focusing mindfully and fully during sexual encounters, breathing to focus during sex, soul gazing, and experimenting with all kinds of touch. But, there is much more to Tantric sex than this, including Tantric sex exercises and couples Tantric sex retreats. One quick Tantric tip, for example, is to purposefully slow your breathing down as you approach orgasm, which is the opposite of what most women do, which is to breath faster as orgasm approaches. The theory is that the slowed breathing will make the orgasm last longer and be more intense. For more Tantric sex tips and information, a very basic, but very good, place to start is *www.goodtoknow.co.uk/relationships*. This site also has links to workshops and books on Tantric sex. Again, going to Good Vibrations, My Pleasure, or the Sinclair Institute store and entering Tantric sex will yield a variety of products. As just examples, My Pleasure has a Tantric Lovers Game, and the Sinclair Institute has a DVD on Tantric sex.

## Get Out of Your Bed

New places to have sex—besides the bed—are another way to spice up your sex life. Sex outside the bed, such as on the couch, may be an especially useful trick for the tired woman who is ready to fall asleep when she crawls in bed. By moving sex to a different location, the strong association between lying down on the bed and falling asleep is less of an issue.

The options for non-bed sex at home are limited only by the architecture of your home, your comfort, and your privacy. Although one couple I know had sex in their car in the garage while their children were inside watching a movie, most couples say that the only time and place they can have sex with children at home is in their own bed at night when the kids are asleep.

Sex in the middle of the living room, or someplace else in the house, is reserved for when children are not around. One couple I know whose children recently left home told me that "the best thing about having the kids gone is that we can have sex anyplace we want." For couples whose children are permanently or temporarily out of the house, even for an hour or so, the options for non-bed sex at home abound. Examples include on a rug in front of the fireplace, an air mattress on a secluded porch, the closet, the bathtub, or a chair in any room in your house. Simply using the guest bed may perk things up a bit, as it may not have the same associations with sleep as your own bed.

> *The best thing about having the kids gone is we can have sex anyplace we want.*
> —Jill, 62

Places to have sex outside the home are also plentiful. A hotel room or bed and breakfast are great options. Also, remember that sex doesn't mean just intercourse.

### spice *homework*

As you walk around your house, look at it in a new way. Look at it as a place that offers lots of interesting places to have sex. Try to find some that appeal to you besides the bedroom. Do the same as you run errands: Have some fun imagining having sex in different places that you go.

### Make Your Bedroom Alluring

Some experts advise making your bedroom a haven where the only things you do are sleep and have sexual encounters. They recommend that you decorate with lighting and colors that are soothing and sensual. Another idea is to get new satin sheets or spray a perfume or cologne on your current sheets. Perhaps spray a scent that Hyla Cass, author of *Natural Highs*, reports to enhance desire: jasmine, vanilla, or rose. Try to keep the room free from things that distract you or prompt your anxiety. For some this might be pictures of one's parents while for others it might be the pile of bills to pay. Some experts advocate taking the television out of your bedroom, even citing an Italian study in which couples that didn't have televisions in their bedroom were twice as likely to have sex as those who had them as part of their bedroom décor. For those interested in watching erotic movies, this suggestion might be counterproductive. Whatever you do, the key is to make your bedroom inviting for sex.

## spice *homework*

Think about the things you could do to make your bedroom more alluring. If something appeals to you and is feasible and affordable, go ahead and do it.

## Delight Through Your Eyes

Before talking about erotic movies, something that can be an intense turn-on for many women, it is important to understand how they are different from pornography. Social scientists generally classify sexually explicit movies into three categories. Violent pornography is sexually explicit material that portrays and endorses sexual violence. Degrading pornography is sexually explicit material that degrades people, usually women. In these films, women are treated as objects for men's pleasure. There are close ups of sexual organs and sex acts, all devoid of emotional interaction. This type of pornography is generally not appealing to women; only a small minority of women finds the observation of male genitalia erotically stimulating. Many women report having a negative emotional reaction to pornography; rather than turning them on, such visual depictions are often turn-offs, physically and emotionally.

Perhaps because of this, many women don't know that erotica exists and that it can be sexually arousing. Erotica depicts sexual activity, without degradation or violence. Research findings on the effects of exposure to nonviolent erotica are consistent: Both men and women are generally sexually aroused by erotic material and both sexes also generally report engaging in sexual activities (of the variety they are accustomed to engaging in) upon watching erotica. For Roberta, a fifty-one-year-old woman, however, the results were neither small nor short-term. She reluctantly and a bit fearfully tried watching some erotica. "Wow. I never knew," she said. "I haven't felt this horny in years. I had forgotten what it feels like." Roberta had made earlier progress in regaining her sex drive with the first *Four T's* of this treatment program. Still, said Roberta, "This was amazing and instant. I have actually been wet and horny for days, because some of the scenes keep popping in my mind. These movies really flipped a switch for me. I went from no drive to feeling insatiable."

*These movies really flipped a switch for me.*
*I went from no drive to feeling insatiable.*
—Roberta, 51

## WHERE'S THE MOVIE GUIDE?

The only way to find out if watching erotic movies will excite you is to watch them. A fairly safe place to start this exploration is with mainstream movies known for their sexual scenes. In May 2008, *Self* magazine recommended nine mainstream movies with hot sex scenes. These included: *The Other Boleyn Girl*, *Atonement*, *Prime*, *The Notebook*, *Unfaithful*, *Amelie*, *The Thomas Crown Affair*, *Shakespeare in Love*, and *Out of Sight*. Certainly, *Self* magazine is not the only publication to list steamy mainstream movie sex scenes, nor are these nine the only hot movies around. Other steamy sex scenes can be found in *Bette Blue*, *Big Easy*, *Coming Home*, *The Unbearable Lightness of Being*, *Risky Business*, and *Nine ½ Weeks*, to name just a few. One way to find out what movies have good sex scenes is to ask your friends for recommendations. A friend of mine, Haley, loves to watch the love scene from the movie, *Titanic*. She says that the scene where the main characters are making passionate love in the car before the ship sinks is the best demonstration of mindful sex that she has ever seen.

For those of you who want to venture a bit further into erotic movies, a good place to start is almost any movie developed and directed by Candida Royalle. Candida is a former porn star who revolutionized the pornographic film industry with her line of women's erotica. These movies feature complex story lines and sex scenes focused on women's pleasure. You can read more about Candida and her films on her website (*www.candidaroyalle.com*). Candida's films were the ones that turned Roberta on so much. Another client of mine, Lizzy, also experimented with Candida's films and found them to be an intense turn-on, although she said she felt there were scenes in some of the movies that still objectified women.

While for many years, Candida was the only producer of erotic films for women, there are now many more options to choose from. The Sinclair Institute has a second website (*www.Better Sex.com*) which has many of the same products available at the Sinclair Institute Store but with additional content and products, including erotic movies. According to their website, the movies they sell have been screened by sex educators and therapists as being sexually healthy to watch, and have also undergone consumer review. Another sex store, Good for Her (*www.goodforher.com*), gives out a *Feminist Porn Award* each year; the movies that have won this award are described in detail on the store's website. Some of the winners are educational in nature. Others feature women-on-women sex scenes.

### IS MY REACTION NORMAL?

If you are heterosexual and watching lesbian sex scenes arouses you, you are not alone. Many heterosexual women tell me that they become aroused by the sexually explicit scenes in the television series *The L Word*, which features a group of lesbian friends and lovers. In one research study, women were shown films of lesbian eroticism while scientific devices monitored physiological changes. The majority of heterosexual women found these scenes sexually exciting.

Some women find gay male porn arousing—perhaps because of the attractive models and the fact that there is no degradation of women in these movies. Some believe that this accounts for some of the success of the movie *Brokeback Mountain*. Movies featuring gay male sex may not be the best choice for a date night with your husband. Most heterosexual men don't report arousal to gay-male porn, although they do report arousal to heterosexual erotica and to lesbian love scenes.

## WITH OR WITHOUT HIM

Many women find that watching erotic films with their husbands is an excellent way to get the heat going. You can discuss what turned you on, perhaps focusing on a particular scene or two that you found especially arousing; sometimes this type of discussion can intensify the excitement. Or, if you prefer not to talk, you can simply use the sexual excitement generated for a passionate sexual encounter.

Watching erotic films alone is also an option; if you do this, you can use the video for your own arousal or to share the energy it generates by having sex with your husband. I have one client, Tina, who simply feels too inhibited and embarrassed to watch such movies with her husband. But, since he is generally always interested in sex, this isn't a problem. She simply watches a scene or two on her own, and finds herself highly aroused. She then uses this excitement for sex with her husband. She says this works even when she is exhausted.

spice *homework*

Think about whether you want to add erotic movies to your repertoire of spices. If you do, check one out. Perhaps start with a mainstream movie like one of those mentioned above. Or, if you want to venture a bit further, a good place to start this exploration is on Candida Royalle's website.

### Another Delight for Your Eyes: Books

Many women find reading erotic books to be a turn-on. Some tired women find that keeping an erotic book by their bedside is a useful way to perk up for nighttime sex. Others like to read passages out loud with their husbands. Erotic books with short stories are especially good for these purposes, as each story can be read independently in five or ten minutes.

If reading erotica is something that you want to try, a good place to start is with Anaïs Nin. Her books, *Little Birds* and *Delta of Venus*, include several short, erotic stories. Both books are known for their erotic content, as well as for the author's literary genius. Another well-known author is Nancy Friday. Her book, *My Secret Garden*, first published in 1973, brought women's sexual fantasies and erotica to the mainstream public. Both this book (released recently in a twenty-fifth anniversary edition) and her more recent book, *Forbidden Flowers*, are collections of the fantasies of real women. These stories are thus not only titillating to read, but can help women feel less alone about their own fantasies, as well as assist them in learning to fantasize. The Sinclair Institute store also has a collection of erotic stories, some to be read and some to be listened to (i.e., erotic books on CD). Another place to start is to simply browse the shelves of your favorite local bookstore, or go to your favorite online bookstore and search the term "Women's Erotica" and see what comes up.

## A Limitless Variety of Spices

Besides the options already mentioned, there are countless other ways—ranging from the tame to the wild—to add novelty to one's sex life. Some couples like to role-play or act out fantasies. You can meet at a bar and pretend you are just meeting and picking each other up for a one-night stand. You can role-play characters (e.g., the plumber and the housewife; the nurse and the patient), complete with dress-up clothes. You can simply approach your husband for sex in a way you have never approached him before. You can add a new sexual act to your repertoire, such as anal stimulation. You can change the way you perform an already existing act, such as finding a new way to give or receive oral sex. Sometimes just putting on new, silky, or sexy clothes propels you to be more imaginative sexually, or to show a different sexual part of yourself. If you are not used to making love to music, you can put some on. You can pick any music, of course.

### spice *homework*

Give one or two of the ideas discussed (e.g., erotic books, erotic movies, sex toys, lubricants) a try. As you do, keep in mind the framework of the spice rack: Stretch your boundaries a bit but don't do anything that doesn't feel comfortable for you. If you haven't already taken a look around the websites mentioned in this chapter, now is the time to do so. You can do so alone or with your spouse, or first alone and then together. In the latter case, for example, you might say, *"The book I am reading recommends we try some new stuff, and the author recommended a few websites. I looked and some of it seems like it might be fun. I want you to read the chapter where different ideas are suggested. I also want to show you the websites I looked at. I think it would be fun to talk about these ideas and decide what we might want to try together."*

# Sex Routines and Signature Moves

Did you ever wonder what happens in the sex lives of other couples? Despite the myriad ideas presented above, many of the couples I talk with have their own sex practices. They have a pattern of what they do together, which has evolved over time based on what works for them. Some of these are described below to illustrate the great variety of what people enjoy sexually. Remember: What works for one couple might be a turn-off to another. But perhaps knowing this will give you more freedom and comfort to try the ideas presented that appeal to you. Perhaps reading about the sex habits of other couples will also get you more in touch with what you do—and don't—find appealing.

When I asked Jean about what she and her husband generally do sexually, she said, "Oh, you mean our typical sexual song and dance?" When I asked Dianna, she said, "Oh, yes, we have our own routine, complete with our signature move."

According to Dianna, her routine is "conventional." She and her husband sometimes start by kissing while they are standing up, but more commonly both get into bed, with candles lit. She wears a negligee because she says it makes her feel sexy and she likes to have something on that her husband can take off. Her husband is naked from the start. They start out kissing and mutually caressing each other all over. Dianna says she especially likes to feel her husband's back and legs. After a lot of kissing and caressing, and after they are both excited, Diana's husband enters her. They continue to kiss and caress with her husband inside of her. Dianna calls this "the appetizer" and the way "we establish a rhythm and a connection that puts us in synch." Once in synch, Dianna says, "We do our signature move—the flip." Dianna's husband flips her over so that she is sitting on top of him. They put pillows under his head to elevate him a bit, and he stimulates her nipples and breasts. Dianna especially enjoys it when her husband puts his knees up and when he sucks on her nipples. In this position and with this stimulation, Dianna has an orgasm. They then flip back over so he is on top and he then has an orgasm. Dianna says that she and her husband have tried other positions and sexual acts, but they never work as well. "I feel like I am with a stranger. Nothing has the staying power of this choreography."

While Dianna calls this "traditional" it is different than other couple's sexual routines and signature moves. While Dianna's routine doesn't include any oral sex, Debbie and Phil's routine always does. Their routine is oral sex turn-taking, followed by intercourse.

Teri is a sixty-three-year-old woman in an open marriage. She is one of the few people I have known over the years for which this arrangement works. She and her husband have always had an open marriage, with both of them having had several one-time encounters outside of the marriage as well as several long-term sexual partners who they see occasionally. They have also had several threesomes and foursomes over the years. Interestingly, however, their marital sex is routine. They kiss and have foreplay, with both of them touching each other. Her husband likes her to rub his penis both with her hands and against her vagina; she likes him to manually stimulate her clitoris. Sometimes she has an orgasm and then they have intercourse, usually with either her on top (which he prefers) or him on top (which she prefers). If they have intercourse before she has an orgasm, her husband always asks if he can do something for her. Usually she says no. If she doesn't have an orgasm before intercourse, she isn't likely to be interested afterwards.

Katie is one of the rare women who does not like or need a lot of foreplay. She likes what she calls the "wicked position." Her husband enters her immediately, with him on top. They then turn about, so that she is on her hands and knees. She doesn't like to talk, but likes her husband to talk dirty to her while they are having sex in this position, telling her his fantasies or using profane words to describe what they are doing.

For Rebecca and her husband, it is all about foreplay. Rebecca describes her husband as "the best kisser I've ever kissed. For us, kissing is the gateway drug." She says that they start out standing, kiss passionately and then furiously disrobe. They fall into bed, with more kissing, more embracing and more stripping off of clothes. Still she says, "We remain focused on kissing." She says that her husband kisses her from her mouth to her neck to her chest. "We both work the top twenty-five percent for a while" she says. They continue to kiss, with a lot of "moving pelvises without penetration." He then touches her manually and gives her oral sex at the same time. She says, "His hands open me up like an oyster and his tongue opens me up like a flower." She says if she can allow herself to relax, it is amazing every time. She has an orgasm, and then encourages him to "climb back up and have intercourse." Sometimes they don't, and he says that his pleasure is having her orgasm. But, mostly they do have intercourse, in the missionary position, and this is when he will have an orgasm.

Francine and her husband start out hugging and caressing each other's backs. They kiss some, but not constantly and not a lot. After a bit of kissing and caressing, she will lie on her back while her husband stimulates her clitoris and the area around it; he usually uses lubricant. He brings her to orgasm manually and then they have intercourse, usually with either her on top or him on top. Like Teri, she says if she doesn't have an orgasm before intercourse, then she doesn't usually want one afterwards. The exception to this is when she and her husband do what they call the "Dead Doggie" position, which is their signature move. After Francine is highly aroused by manual stimulation, her husband will enter her from behind while she is on her hands and knees. Once he is inside, they both lie flat, placing a pillow under her stomach. They both put their hands under her body. While they have intercourse, her husband caresses her breasts while Francine stimulates herself to orgasm by touching her clitoris.

For sixty-nine-year-old Janice and her husband, no form of intercourse is a featured part of the routine. Like many older couples, she and her husband don't like intercourse anymore. Janice brings her husband to orgasm either manually or orally. He brings her to orgasm manually or with a vibrator. Like Teri and Fran, this works best if Janice has her orgasm first.

While all of these couples have sex during waking hours, another variation is sex in the middle of the night. Seventy-five-year-old Nadine says that when her children were young, she was too tired for sex when she went to bed. But, still, she and her husband would cuddle and spoon all night. They would then often wake up in the middle of the night and "be in the mood from all the closeness." Either she or her husband would wake the other up, and they would "make love and go happily back to sleep."

These real-life sex stories illustrate that there is no typical—and no right or wrong—way to have sex in marriage. What is regular for one couple would be novel for another. What is arousing for one couple might be a turn-off for the other. In the best-case scenario, the sex routines that couples develop are ones that have stood the test of time because they reliably work for both partners. Nevertheless, the spicy ideas presented earlier in this chapter can be used to jazz up your routine.

# Spice Step Wrap-Up

Habituation to a routine can be a source of decreased sex drive and interest. Adding novelty is a way to revive a tired woman's sex drive, perhaps because we seem to be drawn to things that interest us—even when we are exhausted. There are countless ways to add novelty to your sex life including (but not limited to) watching erotic movies, experimenting with a variety of lubricants, reading erotic books, getting in new positions, fooling around in different places, playing with new toys, having a sexy game night, and learning about and trying new sexual acts. The only rule is that no one should ever do anything they find repulsive, painful or uncomfortable. It is possible that you are too tired for sex because you are tired of the sex you are having. Find the energy you are lacking by trying something new!

*Chapter 9*

# Anticipation Is Electrifying: Trysts for Tired Women

*Tryst* is an inherently sexy word. Webster's dictionary defines a *tryst* as "an agreement (as between lovers) to meet." A lover's tryst brings to mind images of intense sexual longing and anticipation, covert meetings, and steamy sex. The anticipation of the tryst and the preparation for it heighten the sexual encounter.

*Spontaneous* is defined in Webster's dictionary as "arising from a momentary impulse." Synonyms include impulsive and instinctive. Dictionary examples include the combustion of a motor and bursts of applause.

Yet, in daily language, the words *spontaneous* and *sex* are often paired together. Spontaneous sex just happens. There is no planning or intentionality. Individuals are swept away by their lust and before they can even consider the idea, they are engaged in an act of passion.

# Longing for a Myth

In our culture, spontaneous sex is what many people think they should be having. "Sex should be spontaneous" is a common reply heard by counselors or anyone else who suggests that one plan for a sexual encounter. Planning is thought of as unromantic and as something that will ruin sex.

Yet, longing for spontaneous sex is longing for a myth, albeit a powerful one that vast numbers in our society buy into. Men seem to be especially prone to adhering rigidly to this false belief. But, there is also a good chance that you may be stuck on this myth as well.

If so, you will talk about the spontaneity of sex in your earlier years. Although perhaps you may have had a few instances of impulsive sex in your day, my guess is that most of the sex you are thinking of with longing was actually planned, anticipated, and orchestrated.

Think back to how it felt to get ready for an evening with your husband before you lived together or got married. You picked out your outfit with great care and with an eye toward looking sexually appealing. Perhaps you planned a seductive meal or music. Likely, you put on your sexiest bra and panties and sprayed yourself with perfume. Throughout the evening, you flirted and touched each other seductively. The sexual tension built, and as it did your anticipation of the evening ending in sex heightened. Sex just didn't catch you unaware: it was premeditated and orchestrated. In fact, you did this so well that this choreographed dance of seduction looked effortless. Built-up passion became confused with spontaneity.

Even sex experts sometimes are confused about spontaneous sex. In one sex self-help book for new parents, the author tells readers that in order to have spontaneous sex they have to be willing to create the opportunity for it. Purposefully creating an opportunity for a sexual encounter is not spontaneity—it is a tryst! Once you realize that good sex is almost always intentional, anticipated, and orchestrated, what fun you can have!

## Surprise Him!

One advice column, written by a man, advocates that women give their guys spontaneous sex. Ideas he recommended included wearing a sexy sundress without any underwear when out on a date, finding a brazen way to make this known, and then finding someplace to have a quickie. This idea entails forethought on the part of the woman, and thus isn't spontaneous sex at all. It's a surprise tryst! A surprise tryst is a sexual encounter orchestrated by one partner that catches the other one unaware.

Early on in our parenting years, I gave my husband a surprise tryst. I booked a hotel room. I hired a sitter under the pretense of going out to dinner. When we got in the car, I said I wanted to drive. A few blocks from our house, I pulled over, blindfolded Glenn, and drove him to the hotel. Once we got there, the scene was all set with the wine, food, candles, music, and bubble bath I had dropped off earlier in the day. We enjoyed several hours of uninterrupted time talking, making love, and taking a bubble bath together. We went home and paid the sitter who asked us how dinner was. We both said it was delicious. It was!

Surprise trysts don't have to be this dramatic. Sometimes they look like ordinary sexual encounters to the husband, although the wife knows otherwise. Surprise trysts of this type are particularly useful when husbands reject the idea of a planned tryst. Marcia, a fifty-two-year-old woman, brought up the idea of scheduling a time for sex, and her husband unenthusiastically and sarcastically said,

"*That's* romantic." Marcia summed up the problem beautifully: "So, while we overworked, exhausted women see it as something to look forward to and a time to reconnect that might otherwise simply not happen, perhaps men see it quite differently!" If Marcia can't get Howard to budge, she may want to take control of the situation herself through surprise trysts. She may plan a time that works for her to seduce Howard, perhaps even on a weekly basis as my client Renee does. Renee has decided that once-a-week sex keeps both her and her husband happy. Renee also knows that for sex to work best, it has to be something she primes herself for and spends time planning—so she does, although her husband Kevin doesn't know this. He is simply content with the fact that Renee initiates sex with him about once a week.

> *Overworked, exhausted women see it [sex] as something to look forward to and a time to reconnect that might otherwise simply not happen.*
> —Marcia, 52

Robert is completely aware that his wife Michelle is doing this, but is content in his illusion of spontaneous passion. Robert and Michelle are in their mid-thirties and came to me for marital issues, including Michelle's low sex drive. When I introduced the idea of trysts, Robert was adamantly opposed. Robert didn't like to plan in general, but planned sexual encounters were a particularly repulsive notion to him. Michelle, on the other hand, took immediately to the idea. She was a planner who lived by her schedule and felt that if she could block out time for sex, it would happen.

She also realized that the planning and anticipation would get her in the mood. Michelle and Robert resolved this impasse by agreeing that Michelle would decide in advance when she wanted to make love and initiate it with Robert. They decided that ideally, Michelle would do this once a week. This worked excellently for both of them.

## It's Sex Time!

Another type of tryst that works for some couples is one in which a consistent day or time is set in advance. Many couples find that knowing that they will be having sex on a designated day relieves tensions. Setting trysts in advance alleviates the tired woman's daily worry that her husband will want to have sex that night and that she may not be able to muster the energy. She doesn't have to feel the anguish and guilt that comes with saying she is too tired. Her husband doesn't have to worry that he is being pushy or inconsiderate. He doesn't have to face the risk of rejection.

Perhaps you recall from the introduction that my husband, Glenn, and I started off with this type of tryst. We picked two times that worked for us each week and made these part of our set weekly schedule. Several friends and clients have also used this tryst method with success. My client, Madeline (on a Tuesday/Saturday schedule) passed the wisdom onto a friend. Also a tired woman, the friend became a convert. She wrote Madeline, "Remember that last batch of 'sensitive' e-mails concerning scheduling aspects of your life not normally subject to scheduling? I'll have you know, it works great. Your therapist was right on the money. Truth IS stranger than fiction!"

Fantasy images don't capture the essence of real life with work, children, and chores. If it isn't on the agenda, it isn't likely to happen. This is why for some tired women, having prearranged, set sex times works well.

### How Many Times?

You jotted down your ideal frequency in the *Time* step. Knowing you and your husband's ideal frequency and being willing to work out something mutually agreeable is important to having this type of tryst work successfully. In a perfect world, you and your husband would be in agreement about the frequency. However, one partner often has one idea and the other partner has a different idea. If this happens, the *Talk* skills will be especially useful. If you can't arrive at a compromise, you might want to consider counseling as an option to help you resolve the differences.

*Night doesn't work because we are too worn out.*
—Lisa, 66

### The Right Time: Not Necessarily Nighttime

Some couples have their trysts at the same day and time each week or month. Some couples decide on when their trysts will occur while having the weekly planning meeting that was suggested in the *Talk* step. Either way, in scheduling trysts, it is important to pick times that you won't be exhausted.

There is interesting evidence that testosterone, which is partially responsible for our sex drive, is at its lowest at night. Between exhaustion and decreased testosterone, bedtime is not the ideal time for many women to have sex. As noted by Jean, "It's hard to find time alone with kids running around, but that's a problem because the only time we have is too late at night for me." To get around this, one couple I know sets their alarm an hour early every Friday morning for their tryst. It helps take them into the weekend connected and relaxed. Another has arranged rides for their son to his weekly Boy Scout troop meeting, giving them an hour and a half at home each Monday after dinner. My clients Lisa and Alex, who no longer have children at home, have a Sunday morning tryst. They get up at a leisurely pace, cook and eat a nice breakfast together, and then go back to bed. They initially tried having a weekly evening tryst but as Lisa said, "Night doesn't work because we are too worn out." Lisa and Alex needed reassurance that this was normal. Like many couples, they had bought into the myth that bedtime was the right time for sex. Once they embraced the notion that the right time was the time that worked best for them, they were able to discover that Sundays were a lovely time for their weekly tryst.

## Get It On This Week!

For some couples, a fixed tryst schedule feels too rigid. Some couples aim to have a tryst during a specified period of time. Sandra and her husband have agreed on a weekly tryst that occurs sometime during each weekend. As their weekend progresses, they look for opportunities to meet for their tryst. Sometimes, when energy levels allow, their tryst is at night after the kids are in bed. Other times it is during the day when both children are occupied. Sometimes their weekend trysts are more scheduled, because they hire a sitter and plan their tryst around this. Occasionally they take their children to the sitter's house and go home and make love. Other times, they go out at night and come home after the kids are asleep for their tryst. A few times they had the sitter come during the day and take the children to the park and to lunch, with explicit instructions on how long to stay away from home. The key to this type of tryst is deciding a frequency within a set time period and looking for, or creating, opportunities to make it happen.

## Grab the Opportunity!

Another type of tryst is the opportunistic tryst. This is where a couple keeps sex on the front burner as an important possible use of any time that they find themselves alone together. Opportunistic trysts are more difficult for tired women in the early stages of recovering their drive. They work best after other types of trysts have built up comfort with and energy for sex again. Opportunistic trysts also are easier for parents of older children than those with young children. It's harder to count on young children being occupied for a set period of time. Still, all of the following can present opportunities for parents of young children: children watching television, children napping, and children playing at friends' houses, to name just a few.

Grace and Peter have a teenage son who is often out in the evenings and weekends. Just about every time he goes out and they find themselves home alone, they openly discuss whether or not this would be a good time for a tryst. They also consider whether other opportunities are likely to present themselves later in the week. If not, they take the opportunity given. They remember that they don't need to be horny to have their tryst, but that taking the time to touch will get them interested. Grace also remembers to use her *Thoughts* techniques to consciously let go of her usual task focus. She changes, "I should pay the bills" to "I'm entitled to take a sex break." Knowing that the later into the evening they wait, the less likely they are to have sex, they also have their tryst at the early end of their teen's departure rather than waiting until they go to bed. They also keep in mind that sex entails more than intercourse. Sometimes they end up deciding to have playtime instead, where one partner pleasures the other exclusively. Sometimes they decide that they won't take the opportunity for sex, but they will spend time together talking, cuddling, or both. Certainly, sometimes they decide their chores or work are the main priority for the moment.

The key to opportunistic trysts is to keep the sexual aspect of your relationship in the forefront. The idea is to always be on the lookout for opportunities and to grab them when they come along. Sometimes the opportunity is a short-lived one, and so the tryst has to be a quickie. Annie says, "Sometimes when we have to have a quickie, I watch a few scenes from a Candida Royalle movie, while Bill brushes his teeth and files his fingernails so he can better touch me." Annie laughingly adds, "This isn't a traditional form of foreplay, but it works for us!" Knowing what works for you and your husband for a quick sexual encounter is important if you want to take advantage of fleeting opportunities that present themselves.

## A Hot Hideaway!

Planned getaways are the perfect opportunity for trysts with no time pressure. While not always feasible due to time, availability of sitters, and expense, they are a wonderful way to reconnect with your sex drive and your husband. Getting away for the weekend can be a wonderfully romantic and sexual experience. Even one night away can be terrific. One couple I know, Kate and Tim, book a room, right in their own town, when they can get coverage for their children. Their favorite is to book a bed and breakfast, and take along a picnic of wine, cheese, bread, and fruit, as well as candles and bubble bath. They stay in their room from arrival until the next morning, eating, talking, cuddling, bathing, and making slow, luxurious love. They report that getting away from home, with all its cues of the chores that need to be attended to, and focusing on each other exclusively is a wonderful way to reconnect. Kate and Tim spend the night away for the specific purpose of having an electrifying tryst. Purposefully dedicating a weekend, or even one night, to having great sex is a splendid way to rekindle your sex drive and revitalize your sex life. In fact, there is even a terrific book focused on helping you do just this; *The Great Sex Weekend* by Pepper Schwartz and Janet Lever provides effective and enjoyable recommendations for planning a weekend tryst, the benefits of which will last long past the weekend itself.

Although they didn't specifically plan for a sex getaway, two women recently told me that they had sex with their husbands for the first time in a very long time on vacation. One had not had sex for two years; the other had not had sex for five years. Kendra planned the sex in advance. She knew this would be a good opportunity and she thought about it, priming her mind well in advance. She orchestrated a surprise tryst with her husband. Helen thought about vacation sex also, but she did so with dread. What if even on vacation she didn't want to have sex? What if it just didn't work anymore? The first night, her husband approached her for sex and she declined; she felt exhausted from the travel. The next night, however, she approached him and they had sex. The next day she and her husband, Paul, felt closer than they had in years. They broke out of their no-sex cycle and began a new cycle where sex led to *Provocative Sex Talk* and *No-End-Goal Touching*, and these led to more sex.

## Reassurance for Common Concerns

One common concern mentioned earlier was the notion that sex should be spontaneous. This chapter has hopefully convinced you otherwise. Two additional common concerns about trysts are the pressure for sex to happen and for it to be good.

That sex always needs to be good is a false notion. All sex is not going to be mind-blowing. Sometimes it will be mundane. Sometimes it will be great for one person and mediocre for the other. Couples that have the best sex life are those that know that quality will vary and that are able to talk about this, learn from it, and laugh about it. Sometimes you might have a tryst, and you just can't get into it. The more trysts you have, the less likely this is to happen and the less a big a deal it will be when it does. If it does happen, talk about it, and perhaps switch gears into playtime or another type of time together. Having the tryst is more important than having it be perfect. Any sex is better than no sex at all, for you and for your marriage.

The second common concern relates to the pressure for sex to happen. Not being horny is not a reason to cancel a tryst: Sexual touch can get you there. But, what if, as asked by Nadine, "you schedule for Saturday night and you have a headache and think you would rather die than have sex?" Certainly, this can happen. You can have a tryst scheduled and something else comes up that is more pressing. I had just finished telling my sister about the *Tryst* step. She loved the idea but just hours afterward she ended up in the hospital. In her recovery she said to me, "There goes the *Five T's* for a while!" Lisa and Alex put their weekly trysts on hold for three months when Lisa was dealing with an illness. Sometimes trysts are postponed for more transitory reasons than the illness of one partner. Perhaps your child has the flu or your refrigerator breaks. Life is filled with many unexpected hassles and some will interfere with a scheduled tryst. Don't keep on postponing trysts for reasons that can truly wait. Make sure that if a tryst has to be canceled, you reschedule it. Make sure your trysts don't fade into the background of your life.

## Don't Go Too Long Without

It's good to have in mind a period of time that is just too long to go without a tryst. Grace and Peter, the couple that has opportunistic trysts when their teen son goes out, found that he was suddenly hanging around at home more often. Three weeks went by, and they could find no opportunity. Grace and Peter have about a two- to three-week limit before it starts to feel too long to have gone without a tryst. They decided that because their life situation had changed, they would need to alter their usual method of grabbing opportunities. Instead, they would need to find a set time they could count on. What length of time feels too long for you to go without a tryst?

## Trysts: The Treatment Program Climax

Trysts are the culmination of all the previous steps in the treatment program you have been working through. Give *Thought* to the tryst beforehand to rev up your sexual motor. *Talk* with your husband both before and during the tryst about your sexual desires. Use *Time* alone and together to have you feeling centered in your own life and closer to your husband. Use both affectionate *Touch* to enhance this closeness and sexually provocative *Touch* to keep your juices flowing between trysts. Remember that spontaneous sex is a myth, and that in actuality, anticipation is enticing! Use whatever type of tryst (surprise, set in advance, or grabbing opportunities) works for you, or use a variety of tryst types. To make your trysts even more alluring, spice them up with novelty. Occasionally add in something new that you feel comfortable with, such as a movie, toy, or lubricant. During the tryst, have mind-blowing sex by shutting off your busy brain and focusing on the sensations in the moment. Have these sensations be sensational because your husband knows that you are a slow cooker and how to heat you up. He knows this because you tell him what you and your hot button need both in general and in the moment. Still, remember that all sex won't be perfect and that any sex is better than no sex at all for your personal and relationship health. Never go too long without a tryst. Keep in mind that the more sex you have, the more sex you will want, and that the more sex you have, the easier it will be to get into the flow of having great sex. Engage in *Provocative Sex Talk* after the tryst to keep the heated memories alive and to reinforce the special secret that you and your husband share. If it is a particularly exciting tryst, add it to your bank of fantasy images that you use in your *Thought* step—and let the wonderful cycle continue.

Think of your Final Homework as a culmination of everything you have learned and all of the changes you have made:

Have a tryst with your husband! Keep having them! Make *tryst* a word you use frequently and a special action you engage in often. Enjoy trysts as a vital and central part of your relationship and life! Have great sex—and keep having it!

# Finding a Good Therapist

If you haven't recovered your sex drive, it may be that self-help books are not the forum for you and that therapy would suit you better. Or, perhaps reading this book has made you aware of deeper problems in your marriage or life. Although having such a realization is difficult, it is a positive step. By admitting that you have a problem and taking steps to do something about it, you are already taking actions to improve your life.

The next step is finding a well-trained therapist. If you believe the issue is mostly within you, start with individual therapy. On the other hand, if the issue is within your marriage, start with marriage therapy. But, don't be too concerned about this initial decision; a good therapist will make an assessment of what is best for you and make recommendations. The initial format of therapy is less important than finding a good therapist who can assess what is going on and together with you, design your therapy accordingly.

Word-of-mouth followed by direct questioning of a potential therapist is the best way to find a good therapist. If you have a trusted neighbor or friend who you know is in therapy and is pleased with her therapy, ask her for this therapist's name and number. If you don't know anyone who is in therapy, ask any or all of the following service providers: your hairdresser, your manicurist, or your massage therapist. Ask them if they have clients who have spoken positively about being in therapy and if they will get the therapist's phone number for you. If you are seeking therapy for sexual concerns, an excellent resource is the American Association of Sex Therapists and Educators (AASECT). A list of certified AASECT providers can be found on their website (*www.aasect.org*). Another option for finding a therapist is to ask your physician, although frankly, from my experience, sometimes physicians refer to therapists who have cultivated them as referral sources and this doesn't always mean that the therapist is a high-quality one. Still, your goal is to get at least one, ideally two or three, names of recommended therapists. In the worst-case scenario, look at your local phonebook and pick out a few therapists who are located nearby. You may want to cross-check your list of names with your insurance company and call only those that are covered. Alternatively, calling a highly recommended therapist who isn't covered by your insurance company can be an effective method for finding a quality therapist who is covered. Therapists tend to be most familiar with the qualifications of their colleagues. A good therapist will give you the names of other therapists that he or she recommends if they can't help you, don't have appointments available, or aren't covered by your insurance company.

Your next step is to call these therapists. A good therapist should be willing to chat with you for a few minutes on the phone to answer your questions and help you determine if he or she is qualified to help you. A therapist who becomes impatient or defensive when you ask questions isn't a good choice.

When talking with therapists on the phone, pay attention to your internal reaction to them. It is important to find a well-trained therapist but the "click" or chemistry that you feel with the therapist is equally as critical. Try to talk with at least two therapists and listen to your instincts about who you would work best with.

Ask potential therapists if they conduct consultation sessions. This is when a therapist meets with a client to help both the therapist and the client determine if they are a good match and if the therapist can provide the needed services. Some therapists won't charge for this consultation session and some will charge only if the client subsequently chooses to work with them. While the therapists that do this are few and far between these days, it is certainly reasonable to ask if this is an option. If consultation sessions aren't available and if your insurance or your finances will cover it, it is worthwhile to see two therapists for one session each. Give them both the same opening line. Where the session goes from there will likely make your choice clear.

Below is a list of potential questions to ask a possible therapist:

1. Have you ever worked with someone with _____?
   (Fill in the issue here, such as low sexual desire; issues about childhood abuse; body-image concerns; lack of sex in a marriage; etc.).
2. What is your training and approach to this type of problem?
3. What is your general therapy style or orientation?
4. Are your services covered by my insurance company? If not, can you recommend any providers who are?

5. What is your degree and license in?
6. Do you provide consultation appointments so we can see if we would work well together?

Look for a therapist who is licensed to practice, be that as a psychologist, counselor, or social worker. Look for a therapist who has training and experience with your issue. Look for a therapist who says or conveys that they take an active approach in therapy. While it is nice to feel understood, having a therapist who does nothing but empathize with your concerns isn't likely to result in change. Quality therapy involves mutually agreed upon goals and a way to evaluate when you have met these goals. Therapy shouldn't be a place where you and the therapist meander around a variety of unconnected topics, or simply talk about "how was your week?" each time. You should receive more than a place to vent: you should receive direction to fix your problems and make your life better.

Although developing trust takes time, it is important that you be open and honest with your therapist. Your therapist can only provide help if you tell the truth about your feelings, thoughts, and behaviors. Therapy is a place where you should be able to speak the unspeakable and to bare your soul. It is a place where you should both feel understood and challenged to make changes in your life. Therapy doesn't always feel comfortable, however. A good therapist will sometimes challenge you and confront you. Even so, you should always feel that your therapist has your best interests at heart. If you aren't making progress in therapy, talk with your therapist about this. A good therapist will be open to hearing your perceptions of how things are going. Finally, if therapy ever feels abusive, leave. While a sex therapist will need to talk with you very explicitly about sex and give you homework to complete outside of the session, sex therapy should never involve doing sexual acts with your therapist or demonstrating sexual acts.

If you are open to the process of therapy and if you find a good therapist, therapy can be life altering.

*Appendix B*

# Additional Resources

Below is a listing of additional resources by topic. While there are certainly many more books and websites available on each topic, those listed are the ones I recommend to clients as excellent starting places. You will also find an occasional explanatory note, such as when a book title is not fully representative of the content or when an author or book is particularly recommended.

## Anger

Lerner, Harriet. *The Dance of Anger: A Woman's Guide to Changing the Patterns of Intimate Relationships.* (New York: Harper Collins, 2005).

Several additional books by Harriet Lerner, all in her "Dance of" Series are also listed below. All are highly recommended.

The *Relaxation and Stress Reduction Workbook,* listed below under Stress Management, also has an excellent chapter on dealing with anger.

## Affairs

Lusterman, Don-David. *Infidelity: A Survival Guide.* (Oakland, CA: New Harbinger, 1998).

Spring, Janis A. *After the Affair: Healing the Pain and Rebuilding Trust When a Partner Has Been Unfaithful.* (New York: Harper-Collins, 1996).

Subotnik, Rona, and Harris, Gloria. *Surviving Infidelity: Making Decisions, Recovering from the Pain.* (Avon, MA: Adams, 1999).

## Body-Image

Cash, Thomas F. *Body Image: An Eight-Step Program for Learning to Like Your Looks.* (Oakland, CA: New Harbinger, 2008).

## Communication: General

Lerner, Harriet. *The Dance of Connection: How to Talk to Someone When You're Mad, Hurt, Scared, Frustrated, Insulted, Betrayed or Desperate.* (New York: HarperCollins, 2002).

Gottman, John, Markman, Howard, Gonso, Jonni, and Notarius, Clifford. *A Couple's Guide to Communication.* (Champaign, IL: Research Press, 1979).

The *Feeling Good Handbook*, listed below under Depression, also has an excellent section on communication skills.

The *Relaxation and Stress Reduction Workbook*, listed below under Stress Management, also has an excellent chapter on assertive communication.

## Communication: Sexual

Klein, Marty. *Beyond Orgasm: Dare to Be Honest About the Sex You Really Want*. (Berkeley, CA: Ten Speed Press, 2002).

## Depression (Overcoming It)

Burns, David. *The Feeling Good Handbook*. (New York: Penguin Group, 1999).

## G Spot

Ladas, Alice Khan, Whipple, Beverly, and Perry, John D. *The G Spot: And Other Discoveries About Human Sexuality*. (New York: Holt, 2005)

## Infertility

Resolve: The National Infertility Association: *www.resolve.org*

## Intimacy and Relationships

Gottman, John and Silver, Nan. *The Seven Principles for Making Marriage Work*. (New York: Three Rivers Press, 2000).

Hendrix, Harville, and Hunt, Helen LaKelley. *Getting the Love You Want: A Guide for Couples (20th Anniversary Edition)*. (New York: Henry Holt, 2007).

Hendrix, Harville, and Hunt, Helen LaKelley. *Getting the Love You Want Workbook: The New Couple's Study Guide*. (New York: Simon and Schuster, 2003).

Lerner, Harriet. *The Dance of Intimacy: A Woman's Guide to Courageous Acts of Change in Key Relationships*. (New York: Harper-Collins, 1989).

Wachtel, Ellen. *We Love Each Other But...: Simple Exercises to Strengthen Your Relationship and Make Love Last*. (New York: St. Martin's Press, 2000).

## Masturbation

Dodson, Betty. *Sex For One: The Joy of Self Loving*. (New York: Crown Publishing, 1993).

## Medical and Hormonal Interventions for Low Desire

Because the research in this area is changing so rapidly, I cannot recommend a specific book on this topic. Instead, I recommend the following websites, which tend to maintain up-to-date information and research in a format that is easy to understand. These websites also have search engines; enter terms such as "low libido," "low sexual desire in women," "women's low libido," or "testosterone treatment for low sexual desire." In addition, the websites listed under Menopause and Women's Health also keep up-to-date information on this topic.

National Women's Health Information Center: *www.4woman.gov*

WebMD: *www.webmd.com*

The Kinsey Institute: *www.kinseyinstitute.org*

## Menopause

Boston Women's Health Collective. *Our Bodies, Ourselves: Menopause.* (New York: Simon and Schuster, 2006).

Northrup, Christiane. *The Wisdom of Menopause: Creating Physical and Emotional Health and Healing During the Change.* (New York: Bantam Books. 2001).

North American Menopause Society: *www.menopause.org*

Dr. Susan Love Research Foundation: *www.dslrf.org*

## Mindfulness and Meditation

Kabat-Zinn, Jon. *Wherever You Go, There You Are: Mindfulness Mediation in Everyday Life.* (New York: Hyperion, 1994).

Kabat-Zin, Jon. *Mindfulness for Beginners (Compact Disc).* (Louisville, CO: Sounds True, Inc., 2006).

The *Stress Reduction and Relaxation Workbook,* listed below under Stress Management, also has an excellent chapter on meditation.

## Mismatched Sexual Desire and Other Sexual Problems

Davis, Michelle Weiner. *The Sex-Starved Marriage: Boosting Your Marriage Libido: A Couples Guide.* (New York: Simon and Schuster, 2003).

This book is written for couples that have mismatched sexual desires, regardless of whether it is the woman or the man who has the lower sex drive.

McCarthy, Barry, and McCarthy, Emily. *Rekindling Desire: A Step-by-Step Program to Help Low-Sex and No-Sex Marriages.* (New York: Brunner-Routelege, 2003).

Despite its title, this book addresses an array of sexual issues including mismatched sexual desire among couples, premature ejaculation, erectile dysfunction, painful intercourse, lack of orgasm, and a variety of other topics.

## Orgasm (Information on and Learning To)

Barbach, Lonnie. *For Yourself: The Fulfillment of Female Sexuality.* (New York: Signet, 2000).

Catrall, Kim and Levinson, Mark. *Satisfaction: The Art of the Female Orgasm.* (Boston: Warner Books, 2003).

Heiman, Julia R., and Lopiccolo, Joseph. *Becoming Orgasmic: A Sexual and Personal Growth Program for Women.* (New York: Fireside, 1992).

> Despite its title, this book also contains help for other sexual issues.

Solot, Doroan and Miller, Marsha. *I Love Female Orgasm.* (New York: Perseus Publishing, 2007)

Komisaruk, Barry R., Beyer-Flores, Carlos, and Whipple, Beverly. *The Science of Orgasm.* (Baltimore, MD: John Hopkins University Press, 2006).

*Sex for One*, listed above under Masturbation, will also help women learn to orgasm.

## Parenting (The Early Years)

Gottman, John Mordechai and Gottman, Julie Schwartz. *And Baby Makes Three: The Six Step Plan for Preserving Marital Intimacy and Rekindling Romance After Baby Arrives.* New York: Three Rivers Press, 2008).

## Power Issues in Marriage
## (Re-Thinking and Re-Negotiating Them)

Carter, Bette. *Love, Honor, and Negotiate: Building Partnerships That Last a Lifetime.* (New York: Simon and Schuster, 1997).

Schwartz, Pepper. *Love Between Equals: How Peer Marriage Really Works.* (New York: Simon and Schuster, Free Press, 1995).

## Sexual Abuse and Rape (Recovery from)

Bass, Ellen and Davis, Laura. *Courage to Heal: A Guide for Women Survivors of Child Sexual Abuse 20th Anniversary Edition.* (New York: HarperCollins, 2008).

Davis, Laura. *The Courage to Heal Workbook: A Guide for Women Survivors of Child Sexual Abuse.* (New York: HarperCollins, 1990).

Haines, Staci. *The Survivor's Guide to Sex: How to Have an Empowered Sex Life After Child Sexual Abuse.* (San Francisco: Cleis Press, 1999).

Dealing with one's sexuality as a survivor of childhood sexual abuse is generally an issue that is dealt with later in recovery. This resource is included for abuse survivors who are at this stage of their recovery and healing.

Matsakis, Aphrodite. *Rape Recovery Handbook.* (Oakland, CA: New Harbinger, 2008).

## Sex Education and Information

Johanson, Sue. *Sex, Sex and More Sex*. (New York: Harper Collins, 2005)

Talk Sex with Sue website: *www.talksexwithsue.com*

## Sex Manuals

Joanides, Paul. *Guide to Getting it On!* (Waldport, OR: Goofy Foot Press, 2001).

Winks, Cathy, and Semans, Anne. *The Good Vibrations Guide to Sex: The Most Complete Sex Manual Ever Written*. (San Francisco: Cleis Press, 2002).

## Stress Management

Eshelman, Elizabeth Robbins, McKay, Mathew, and Fanning, Patrick. *The Relaxation and Stress Reduction Workbook*. (Oakland, CA: New Harbinger, 2008).

This is one of my all-time favorite self-help books. It contains straightforward and effective exercises to relieve stress. It has chapters on a variety of stress management techniques, such as deep breathing and self-hypnosis, as well as chapters on refuting negative thoughts, meditation, anger management, time management, assertion, nutrition, exercise, workplace stress, and other useful topics for busy and stressed women.

## Time Management

The *Stress Reduction and Relaxation Workbook*, listed above under Stress Management, has an excellent chapter on time management.

## Vulvodynia

National Vulvodynia Association: *www.nva.org*

## Women's Health (Including Sexual Health)

Boston Women's Health Collective. *Our Bodies, Ourselves: A New Edition for a New Era*. (New York: Simon and Schuster, 2005).

Boston Women's Health Collective Website: *www.ourbodiesourselves.org*

## Women's Sexuality (Including Sexual Dysfunction and Enhancing Sexual Relationships)

Berman, Jennifer and Berman, Laura. *For Women Only: A Revolutionary Guide to Reclaiming Your Sex Life*. (New York, Holt, 2005).

Berman, Laura. *Real Sex For Real Women: Intimacy, Pleasure, and Sexual Wellbeing*. (New York: DK Publishing, 2008).

## Books for Your Husband (To Help Him, Educate Him, or Assist Him in Being a Better Lover)

Zilbergeld, Bernie. *The New Male Sexuality: The Truth About Men, Sex, and Pleasure.* (New York: Bantam Books, 1999).

Kerner, Ian. *She Comes First: The Thinking Man's Guide to Pleasuring a Woman.* (New York: HarperCollins, 2004).

This book is focused mainly on oral sex. Still, I find that even the title can help get men thinking about the idea of the woman having an orgasm before intercourse, something which was discussed in this book. A companion book by this same author, *He Comes Next,* is also a great resource for women on male sexuality and pleasuring men.

McCarthy, Barry, and Metz, Michael. *Men's Sexual Health: Fitness for Satisfying Sex.* (New York: Routledge, 2008).

# Index

# About the Author

Laurie B. Mintz has a PhD in counseling psychology from The Ohio State University and is licensed as a psychologist in both Missouri and California. She has maintained a private practice counseling women and couples for more than twenty years. She has taught at the University of Southern California and the University of Missouri–Columbia, where she is currently a tenured professor. She has published extensively in professional psychology literature, with more than 100 articles, book chapters, and conference presentations to her credit. She has also appeared regularly in the popular media, providing information and expertise on topics pertaining to women's mental health, including body-image, eating disorders, stress-management, couple issues, and sexuality. Dr. Mintz is married and the mother of two teenage daughters. She resides in Columbia, Missouri, where, thanks to following her own advice, she enjoys a passionate and satisfying sexual relationship with her husband of twenty-four years.